12 Steps **to** Raw Foods

How to End Your Addiction to Cooked Food

Victoria Boutenko

Raw Family Publishing

Raw Family Publishing
2253 Highway 99 North, #58
Ashland, OR 97520, U.S.A.

www.RawFamily.com

Photography on the front cover by Dragomir Vukovic

Edited by Jane C. Picknell

Cover and interior design by Lightbourne

Library of Congress Catalog Card Number 2001118915

ISBN 0-9704819-3-4

Disclaimer: The information contained in this book is not intended as medical advice. Victoria Boutenko does not recommend cooked foods or standard medical practices. The authors, publishers and/or distributors will not assume responsibility for any adverse consequences resulting from adopting the lifestyle described herein.

While the 12 Steps, identified were inspired by the Twelve Steps of A.A., they are not really an adaptation. Rather, they were created specifically for this publication, and should not be construed otherwise. A.A., which is a program concerned only with recovery from alcoholism, and is not in any way affiliated with this publication

I dedicate this book to Donald O. Haughey without whose encouragement this book would not be possible.

Acknowledgements

I thank all my dear friends throughout the world
who inspired me to present thinking.

I thank all Editors, Readers and Artists
for their kindness and patience.

Special thanks to
Donald O. Haughey and
Elizabeth and David Bechtold
for financing my book.

CONTENTS

Foreword

by Gabriel Cousens

Twelve Steps to Raw Food is a breakthrough work for the live food movement. The breakthrough is the understanding, humbly articulated by Victoria Boutenko for the first time, that there are many people who are literally addicted to cooked food. Because of this addiction to cooked food they have a very difficult time transitioning gracefully to a full live food diet. This book is an answer to their problems. Victoria, in a very thoughtful and compassionate way, outlines a breakthrough 12 Step program to support people successfully in their transition to live foods. She takes much of her understanding about the idea of cooked food addiction from the tradition of 12 Step programs. Starting with this as a base, she has formulated a very compassionate system for helping people make a successful transition to live foods.

As a holistic physician, psychiatrist, family therapist, and a person on 100% live foods since 1983, and who has been helping thousands of people shift towards live foods, this book provided me with a tremendous new insight. In my own life, my transition to live foods was motivated by an intense spiritual focus and my transition was done without the help of others or much knowledge. I was personally fortunate in that I never really experienced the difficulties of addiction. Because of this, I simply didn't have this insight to help understand the difficulties that many of my clients were having making the transition to live foods. At the Tree of Life Rejuvenation Center, a live food rejuvenation center in Patagonia, AZ, where I am director, we incorporate many of the steps Victoria talks about for helping clients succeed with live foods, but not with the clarity that she creates in this book. Yes, we teach Step 2, that vegan live foods are the dietary blueprint for the coming age of peace; and yes, we teach Step 3, the basic skills, raw recipes, and equipment use; we share Step 4, compassion and tolerance for people who eat cooked food; Step 5, of how to avoid temptation; Step 6, creating support groups; Step 7, finding alternative activities to eating; we address Step 8, personality repatterning and Step 9, the psychology of food addiction, giving healing techniques and processes with a special course called Zero Point for overcoming these food addictions; Step 10, we show people to trust their intuition with food; encourage and inspire Step 11, the joy of spiritual awakening in our function as a spiritual sanctuary, and Step 12, we encourage the general growth of the live food movement, giving support with books, and even offering a live food University Master's Degree course. But, we missed the punch line, Step 1, helping those with difficulties to realize their uncontrollable addiction to cooked foods and the actual need for a formal 12 Step approach! Step 1 gives power to all the other steps.

This breakthrough makes this book so valuable and clear.

It is this crystallization of this potent issue in the live food movement that I personally didn't quite understand until I began talking to Victoria about it and had an opportunity to read her book. I applaud Victoria and this book—for this breakthrough. I am very happy that this book is on the market. I will be recommending this book to my clients that come to the Tree of Life. It speaks to a problem that perhaps not everyone has, but that many, many people do have. I believe that it will provide a vocabulary, understanding and a compassion that will serve many people.

Victoria, by sharing the stories of her own transition and difficulties and that of her family, makes it a very personable book. Her anecdotes give people something concrete and human that people can identify with. Her genuine humbleness makes this book even more powerful. The stories of her family's transition, of their struggles, and of the growth that they all experienced in this process, are an inspiration. The reading of this book for many people is really a reading of their own struggles and a solution, or at least a pathway, to success.

Although the most important contribution to this book is the clean, clear insight that for many people, cooked food is an addiction, Victoria gives a very solid overview of the importance of live foods for our health and our well being. She also shares insights into food preparation that are foundational and, in my opinion, are absolutely perfect in terms of getting people to understand that it's not about the recipes but about understanding and playing with food in a way that encourages us to make our own creations in the simplest ways to meet our needs. As I read her book I really appreciate her sophisticated understanding of the ins and outs of the transition to live foods. For example, she makes the point that raw food has to be delicious, particularly in the beginning, because people need the psychological comfort of gourmet quality to make the transition. At the same time pointing out that once people are more involved in the live food way of life, there's less need for the gourmet level. She gives people gems to which they can hang on to help them to be very successful in becoming raw food people.

Perhaps one of the most important elements is her compassion that comes through in her writing based on her own experiences and that of her family. She helps us look at the cultural attachments, social pressures, the programming from birth, the addictive quality of particularly the processed food, and artfully gives people ways to deal with all of these issues.

Another aspect that makes this book very positive for people is its support for turning people into their own best expert. There's a lot of confusion in all fields involved in nutrition, whether it's live foods or not. And her clear way of approaching this is encouraging people, once they're through the detoxification, to trust their own body cravings because these cravings often tell a person what they really need for their bodily health at that moment. Another aspect to her work is a very excellent chapter on detoxification as part of the transition to healing. She skillfully covers all the symptoms that people commonly have and turns the detox into a celebration. In fact, she turns this whole transition process, which for so many people is not the easiest thing, into a celebration – a celebration of life and of love for ourselves.

This book is destined to become a classic. I am grateful for the opportunity to write an introduction and I strongly recommend it to anyone who is helping others move into a live food lifestyle, to any teacher of live foods, and to any live food friend who needs support at any level. This book is one of the most supportive and nurturing offerings in the live food movement that I've seen in years. Victoria Bountenko has made a wonderful contribution with this book. I am grateful for this breakthrough!

Blessings to your health, well-being, and spiritual joy,

Gabriel Cousens, M.D., M.D. (H)
Director of the Tree of Life Rejuvenation Center, author of
Conscious Eating and *Spiritual Nutrition and The Rainbow Diet.*

A Note from the Author

Dear Reader,

I believe that you cannot remember **my** thoughts or **my** words. You can remember only your own thoughts that you have while reading or listening. Then these are your own discoveries, and you shift yourself in your own way. That is why when I teach classes I always create a dialogue. I form some key questions and ask my audience to give me honest answers.

I will be asking you too, my reader, some important questions in this book as if you are in my class. I feel that to be honest is important for you. Not for me, because many of you I will never see. Please be as honest as you can. And I promise to be as honest as I can. This way we will have a dialogue. A sincere dialogue is the best way to follow the truth.

When I say in my classes that cooked food is addictive, people laugh. When I say we should have "Cooked Food Anonymous," people laugh even more. But in fact this is not funny. Most people go on raw food for some serious reasons, like me, my husband and my children. To me going on raw food meant choosing life over death. I was dying, I went on raw food and I am alive, healthy and happy. I am grateful that I had support from my family. When I was watching other people trying to be raw fooders, I have found that staying on the raw food diet is difficult without support. When we go on raw food, we are acting against everything that is considered normal and expected around eating.

Out of compassion to all people who experience difficulties staying on a raw food diet, with the support from my family, I have created this 12 Step program. I tried it for one year in many classes before putting it into a book. I have been teaching 12 Steps to Raw Food, that treats cooked food as an addiction. Students who have taken this program are staying successfully 100% raw. They are experiencing no temptation to eat cooked food. Just none. These 12 Steps help people to stay on raw food, no matter what. They work! Now, using this program, people are organizing their own weekly support groups. They study 12 Steps to Raw Food in Seattle, Eugene, Silver Spring, San Mateo and many other cities. These groups are growing every day. If you want to contact them please see the information in the end of this book.

We wanted to try this program longer before publishing this book, but we received such an avalanche of requests from all over the world for it, that we decided to publish the book now. We will continue to work on the 12 Step program and are planning to publish a more complete edition in the future.

In Part One of this book, we will discuss why eating raw food is the most healthy and nutritious way to eat. In Part Two we will explore how to stay on the raw food diet using the 12 Steps to Raw Food program.

PART ONE

Why Eat Raw?

CHAPTER ONE

Life and Energy

When people talk about raw food, they usually talk about enzymes. Enzymes are energy. Enzymes are life. We cannot see enzymes with our naked eye, but we can see the life and energy that is the result of enzymes. For example, if I take two almonds, one raw and one roasted, and plant them in the soil, within three weeks the roasted almond will have disintegrated into the soil. The raw almond will remain where I planted it. In spring the snow melts on the mountain and flows down to water the soil, inhibitors will be unlocked in the almond and it will have the potential to give birth to a beautiful big almond tree, which will give birth to thousands more beautiful almonds. As this illustration shows, the difference between the roasted almond and the raw almond is life and death. One has enzymes and one does not. One carries within the potential of life, the other has had life cooked out. If I were to take two almonds (one raw and one roasted) to a scientist and ask for an analysis of both almonds, the scientist will see no nutritional difference between the two almonds. Both almonds have the same amount of calcium, potassium, sodium, magnesium, zinc and copper as if they are absolutely equivalent nutritionally. However, as the example shows, one carries life in enzymes while the other does not.

In order to understand better how enzymes work, let us fantasize a story. On a beautiful June day you are walking through an apple orchard. You look for apples, but they are still green and hiding in the leaves. You cannot see them easily and they don't really smell. You return to the orchard in July. The apples are big and red and they smell great. The apples seem to be calling to you, "See me, smell me, eat me." You realize that to an apple, being eaten by an animal or a human being means the continuation of life. You reach out and pick a large red apple. You take a bite. The apple is filled with live enzymes. As you enjoy the flavor and texture of the apple, the enzymes (likened to little handy-men with suitcases full of magic healing tools) work on your body. As you walk along, the enzymes work through your body as a healing team, repairing what needs attention. You feel good and full of energy because the apple carries the enzymes within it to digest itself. Your body does not have to put out extra effort to digest the apple. Later the apple leaves your body in the form of fertilizer and continues to live. You have participated in the circle of life. Everything is circular. It is a universal law.

The following weekend you return to the orchard and pick a basket of apples. You take the apples home to make baked apples with caramel and cinnamon, just like your grandmother used to make. You create your dish and put it into the oven to cook. The baked apple looks pretty and smells delicious. It looks as nutritious as that apple you picked and ate raw last weekend. But it is not. This apple has been cooked and the enzymes are destroyed.

You bite into the sweet baked apple, caramel and cinnamon stimulate your taste buds creating a pleasant sensation. You finish your serving and then go to lie down. You are feeling a little sluggish and tired. Inside your body your own enzymes have to leave their work, maybe cleaning the liver, protecting you from tumors and evacuating toxins here and there, to come digest the cooked apple that does not have any enzymes of its own. When this apple finally leaves your body, into the toilet, it is filled with your own enzymes. These enzymes are gone forever. Cooked food does not contain live enzymes and so takes enzymes from your body to digest the food. These enzymes then leave your body, leaving you with fewer enzymes than you started with. Dr. Edward Howell, a leading nutritionist, suggested that the average American at the age of 40, has only 30% of their enzymes left. We can still walk, talk and think at this point, but when we have only 30% of our enzymes left, plus they have to give about 75% of their energy to detoxify the body, we become less sensitive to other people, and to ourselves. We may survive physically but not spiritually.

The good news is that even if we have only 30% of our enzymes left, we still can live our portion of life, if we go on a raw diet and let the body purify itself.

There is a lot of misunderstanding and confusion in the field of enzymes. In fact many licensed nutritionists don't understand the importance of enzymes in our food. If you want to have a proper diet, gaining complete clarity about enzymes is crucial. For example, let's look at the difference between raw fat and cooked fat. Why does fat exist? We all need fat to lubricate our eyes so we can see, to lubricate our skin so it is soft and to lubricate our hair. We need fat to lubricate our joints, so whenever we move our joints we don't squeak like an old garage door. We can't get live fat from pasteurized milk, butter, sour cream or roasted nuts because it is all cooked! We could be very obese but lack real fat. Our bodies are desperate for raw live fat. The best sources of live fat are avocado, young coconut, durian, olives, nuts, seeds and cold pressed extra virgin olive oil.

I remember when I was very obese. I was 120 pounds more than I am now. During that time I started to crave avocados. I was able to eat eight avocados a day. Before that, to me, they tasted like soap. When I was eating avocados, I started to lose weight faster. This is because the enzyme in the fat of avocados, lipase, was able to penetrate my saturated fat deposits, break them into smaller pieces, and take them out of my body. Isn't that amazing?

Another example is calcium. When we lack calcium, we are advised by advertising to drink pasteurized milk. You've all seen the ads that ask "Got Milk?" I would argue that when we need calcium, the more appropriate question is to ask "Got wheat grass?" or "Got sesame seed milk?" Cow's milk is not intended for human consumption; it does have calcium, but it also contains very concentrated protein and produces excessive mucus. Secondly, pasteurized milk has been heated until the enzyme activity has stopped. The enzymes are destroyed; there is no life. The body only absorbs empty lifeless shells of calcium molecules.

Wheat grass is where a cow gets her calcium and is easy digested by the human body because the molecule of chlorophyll and the molecule of human blood are almost identical.

Sesame seeds are the richest in calcium among all other seeds and nuts. Sesame milk is delicious and can easily replace cow's milk.

As I said earlier, enzymes are life and energy. We are human beings and we are spiritual beings. We need energy so we move and work and also love, share, communicate and be sensitive to each other. Every time we eat cooked food we loose enzymes. In our cooked food filled bodies, our enzymes are doing hard work. Because cooked food does not have enzymes, our body cannot use it. Therefore, the body treats cooked food as a toxin and is only concerned with getting rid of it.

Can we replenish lost enzymes? There are different opinions on that. Dr. Howell says that all living creatures have a fixed enzyme potential and cannot replenish them. Often people ask if they could replenish their enzymes with supplements. I believe we cannot. The enzyme supplements that are sold in the store are nothing but dehydrated raw food. For example, the supplements sold to help digest cooked beef steak are made of raw dehydrated beef liver. I understand that the cooked beef steak has a different nutritional content than the raw dehydrated beef liver.

Can we eat a lot of apples and store up the enzymes? I believe that we cannot take the enzymes from an apple and keep them in our body. They enter our body and do some work while they are there, but they don't stay there. This is my opinion based on my reading and experience, but no one yet knows the exact truth about replenishing enzymes. I can tell you that I rebuilt my own health not because I got enzymes from outside, but because I preserve my own enzymes by not eating cooked food. My enzymes are no longer overloaded with the work of digesting cooked food and I experience radiant health and an abundance of energy.

I also believe that if we follow our heart and do what we are meant to do with this life, then we become dedicated spiritual beings, and we can be granted an extra portion of energy from the universe.

CHAPTER TWO

The Human Body Never Makes Mistakes

We each need to trust our own body. I encourage you to follow your own intuition, your own feeling and your own experience. I do not want you to do anything because I say so. We are each unique individuals with different body needs. We need to be our own best expert. If you change your diet because Victoria says so, it won't last. Or, it may only last until the next "expert" presents you with a different idea on health. I suggest that you do something only because you feel it is right for you.

There are many good teachers in the world today. Let's imagine following each suggestion every good teacher makes. One nutritionist advises us to avoid eating fruits, because fruits have sugar that can lead to cancer. Another popular nutritionist advises us to eat only fruits and no vegetables. Yet another argues that nightshades and citruses will cause arthritis in our body and will ruin our bones. Dr. Hilton

Hotema, who lived to be 100 years old, tells us not to eat green cabbage, kale or greens because they are from the opium family and are toxic. Another nutritionist has written a new sprouting book in which she states that sprouts are so toxic not even animals will eat them. Another brilliant man and a good friend of mine, warns us not to eat grains as they cause brain damage. Hygienists tell us not to eat nuts or dried fruits because "it is concentrated food." I heard another popular teacher of raw foods say not to eat carrots, turnips or roots because they are hybrids and the body does not recognize them as food. If we follow the advice of all of these good teachers, do we have anything left to eat? Instead of a raw fooder I could become breatherian (one who lives by only breathing the air). How confusing. The only solution is to listen to your own body.

Let's do an experiment. If you went to an organic fruit stand right now and picked out one fruit, what would it be? A pear, apple, orange, fig, papaya, banana, grape, avocado, mango or cherry? Is everyone reading this book picking the same fruit? Probably not. We are all individuals. Your body knows what you need. Whatever fruit you choose, that is what your body is ordering from you today. Your job is to get your body what it needs. Tomorrow your body may want the same fruit or something new. Let your body lead.

I've been following my body for eight years. During this time I have attended many excellent lectures where the speakers have argued against eating one type of food or another. I remember one teacher arguing against eating grains. That day I was craving quinoa, so I said to the speaker, "I appreciate your opinion and your research, but my body is my boss." When my body says it wants quinoa, I sprout it and eat it. What else could I do? I need to follow my body. My body knows best. Listen to your body and your intuition for health and happiness.

Please believe in your own intuition and don't make the mistake of thinking that someone else knows better about your body than you do. Your body is so beautiful and so wise. Every cell of the 35 trillion cells in your body has its own soul and its own wisdom and knows what to do. Let's imagine that a piece of dust is falling into your right eye. Which eye will blink? Your right eye, of course. Your left eye won't blink by mistake, because your body never makes mistakes. Your mother gave birth to a perfect baby. Our bodies are perfect. When we start bossing our bodies around and not listening to our own wisdom, we get into trouble. For example, what is the standard response to fever in our culture? Aspirin. Right. I believe that if my body has created a fever, then I need a fever. When the body creates diarrhea, the body is saying I need diarrhea. Taking medication to stop the diarrhea is working against the wisdom of the body. Our body never makes mistakes. We all know what we need to do if we listen to our body.

When my family had been on raw food for two months, my children began craving different fruits. Sergei asked for mangoes and blueberries and Valya asked for olives and figs. The kids' cravings were so strong, I had to hustle to keep up with them. For example, I gave Sergei a mango. He ate it and wanted more. I bought him a whole case of mangoes thinking that would last him a week. He sat down and ate the entire case in one day, skin and all. He then said "I wish there were more mangoes," so I bought him another case. The same thing happened with blueberries. I bought him a two-pound bag of blueberries and he ate it in one sitting. Valya liked figs. She'd ask for fresh figs, dry figs, black figs. She could never have enough figs; she also liked eating olives. During our travels that spring, we visited our friend Marlene. Marlene had a beautiful olive tree. There were olives underneath the tree already starting to rot. Valya said, "I want to try them. Oh, they are delicious." I tried them. To me they were too bitter. Valya enjoyed the olives so much that she gathered them up in plastic bags to take with us.

The next stop on our trip was a visit to Dr. Bernard Jensen, a world famous clinical nutritionist. We asked Dr. Jensen what Sergei needed to eat for diabetes. He looked in his books and told us that the best thing for diabetes is mangoes and blueberries. Wow. Then we asked him what Valya needed to eat to help her asthma. He said figs and olives. I told him that was exactly what our children were asking for. Then Dr. Jensen asked me what my cravings were. I told him that I didn't know because I always was eating what was on sale.

I understood then that our bodies crave certain foods because of need. Our children's bodies talked to them sooner than our adult bodies. After several more weeks, Igor and I developed cravings. I remember one day when I had a scallion attack. I suddenly sensed scallions everywhere. I looked at the green wallpaper, and I thought, "I want scallions." I went to the store and bought ten bunches of scallions. I craved scallions so strongly that by the time I got to the cash register, I had only nine bunches remaining. I couldn't explain to the surprised cashier why I had eaten an unwashed bunch of scallions between the produce section and check out. I paid for the scallions, including the ones I'd eaten, and left the store, leaving a puzzled cashier staring after me. I went home, mixed the scallions with avocados and ate them all in one sitting. I called and asked Dr. Jensen what he could tell me about my scallion attack. After all, I had read that hygienists say not to eat onions or garlic because they irritate our mucus membranes. Dr. Jensen told me that sometimes when people have a lot of mucus their body craves something like onions that will help to dissolve the mucus and bring it out.

Have you ever craved sweets? When our body needs calcium, we actually crave sweets. Calcium, in nature, has a sweet taste. If we plant strawberries on a soil rich in calcium, the strawberries will be very sweet. Sometimes we are so low in calcium that we become addicted to sweets. I had a hard time getting off sweets. I did not eat them, but every time I went in the store I had to cover my eyes so I wouldn't see them while on my way to the produce section. If I looked at the sweets I suffered from wanting to go and try them. I shared with a friend how much I craved sweets. He said, "Victoria, you are just craving calcium." He told me to soak sesame seeds and make sesame milk and drink it every day for two weeks on an empty stomach.

I followed his instructions. First, I made sesame milk from sesame seeds with honey. In a few days I didn't want it to be as sweet, so I added less honey. After a week I didn't want honey at all. Then I wanted a bitter taste, so I switched to brown sesame seeds. For two weeks I didn't go anywhere without my big mug of sesame milk. Two weeks later another friend offered me a medjool date. I love medjool dates! I took one bite and I could not swallow it! It was too sweet for me. The balance in my body had changed. I didn't want sweet things anymore, not even good sweet things. Fantastic!

Grapes were in season that summer and I didn't want grapes. Sesame milk is the champion of calcium.

When Sergei broke his clavicle, the first thing he craved was wheat grass juice, and the second thing he craved was sesame milk. I came home after being gone all day to Valya saying "Talk to him! He's exploiting me! He's forcing me to make him sesame milk every 30 minutes! I cannot do anything! I cannot do my homework, I cannot go and play, I have to make sesame milk all day long for this guy!" Because Sergei had a broken clavicle, he was craving sesame milk. When he healed, he didn't need physical therapy. We were told by doctors that it would take about eight to twelve weeks for Sergei to heal, but Sergei healed much more rapidly than that because of the sesame milk. In only two weeks Sergei's body grew the calcified ball which causes the bones to grow together so they can begin to heal.

If you don't know what your body is craving, you'll do what Valya used to do. She'd open the fridge, and defrost it standing there, wondering "What do I want?" She couldn't find anything that she wanted, so she'd close the fridge. She knew she wanted something, but she just didn't know what. Sometimes you, too, will crave something you have never tried in your life. You'll look at the array of food offered and nothing will look appealing, because you crave something that's not there.

To help you identify cravings, you can start buying fruits and vegetables that you have not tried yet. What works very well for one person doesn't always work for everyone. Once I was supposed to make lunch for 25 people. I went out into my yard and suddenly the dandelions looked so yummy. So I decided to try one. The dandelions tasted sweet to me. They were not bitter at all. I took a big bucket and I filled it with the dandelions. I told my guests that we were having a very special lunch. I put six avocados and lemon juice into the food processor to make a dressing. I poured the dressing over the dandelions and mixed with my hands and my love. I put this piece of art on the table. My guests tried my new dish and exclaimed, "This is so bitter!" I ended up eating my new creation all by myself. The next morning I woke up and my skin was all yellow. My dish created a great liver cleanse. Before the dandelion cleanse, my skin was white and pasty. Since that dandelion feast I have rosy cheeks. My body knew I needed dandelions.

The human body is so beautiful, yet we take our body for granted. I want to tell you a few things about our miraculous body. I was told in school that blood is something like red paint; it floats in our body because of gravity pushing down, and then the heart pumps it back up, and it keeps flowing down, and it pumps it back just like red paint. No! Blood is not red paint. Blood is a miraculous river of life that travels through trillions of vessels at cosmic speed. It does not just flow because of gravity. Blood goes in any direction necessary according to the universal laws that we cannot even understand. When I cut my finger, the blood washes the dirt out. Then the blood clots and seals the wound. The blood forms a scab and when this scab peels off, I have new skin where the cut was.

The human body is so fascinating. Take our hand for example. The hand consists of 27 very intricate bones. My hand can grab an apple, peel a banana, pull roots from the ground or help me to climb a tree. When I put my hand in the water, the water does not penetrate the skin, yet if my body needs to sweat, I can sweat through my hand that just a minute ago seemed waterproof. Our bodies are so miraculous that we have to be fascinated and thankful for every single hair we have on our head (before we lose it)!

Our body wants us to be beautiful. Every single person's body wants to be beautiful and healthy. What stands in the way of the body? I once thought that I had bad luck because I was born with an ugly body. I once thought that my body was just horrible. It always treated me with pain and pimples, and whatever I ate, I gained weight. Since I've been on raw foods, I've lost 120 pounds. I have more energy than I ever had in my life. Now I can run and jump and play. I love my body. Yet, this is the same body that I had eight years ago. The same body that I thought was ugly and causing me pain. The same body that I thought I was just unlucky to get. What changed? I got my "headucation" out of the way. I started listening to my body instead of my head. I eat raw foods because that's what my body needs. The only insurance to be healthy is to learn what your body wants and needs. Our bodies want us to be beautiful and healthy. All we need to do is listen to our body's intuition, and then follow.

CHAPTER THREE

The Law of Vital Adjustment

The body of every living thing is dedicated to the survival of the owner or spirit that lives within. The body does everything to protect itself and to keep the species going, no matter what the obstacle. If the body has two choices, to be hurt and possibly killed or to survive, it will always choose survival. This is called the vital law of adjustment. We have several examples of this adjustment.

Every living thing adjusts to its environment. For example, rabbits change their fur from brown in the summer to white in the winter. The purpose of the change in fur color is to camouflage the rabbit in the fields in summer and the snow in winter. This camouflage increases the chances of the rabbit's survival against predators. If we jump into a very hot shower in the morning, we are likely to get scalded. If we get into the shower with moderately hot water, and then turn up the water gradually, we can make it really hot without feeling discomfort. The human body adjusts to the gradual increase in temperature and we don't get burned. After spending the winter in shoes, our feet hurt when walking bare foot on gravel in the spring. Yet, by the end of summer, our feet have toughened up and it's easy and pain free to walk on gravel. The micro muscles in our feet have become stronger and, when stepping on the gravel, the foot curves against and around the gravel. The body has adjusted to take care of us. Or has this ever happened to you? One day you are driving through the big city and you get stuck in a traffic jam. You turn on the radio to help pass the time. The next morning you get up early for work and very quietly go to your car, turn the key in the ignition, and auugh!! The music is so loud it hurts your ears. How did this happen? The answer is interesting. When you were in the city, your hearing adjusted to the noise of the traffic. You actually became deaf, perhaps by 20%. Your body made this adjustment because noise is very harmful and if the body doesn't adjust you could get a headache. Your body adjusts to the noise and then you go home to the quiet neighborhood and sleep. Your body now readjusts to the quietness of your home, however, your car doesn't.

If you go to Russia, the men there drink a bottle of vodka a day. They sell vodka next to the bread; it is considered part of the diet. If we find someone who never drank alcohol like a healthy child or Australian aborigine vegetarian, and we give him/her just one glass of vodka, this person could die of alcohol poisoning. Russian men, on the other hand, have bodies that have adjusted to the ingestion of alcohol. In the book *Man's Higher Consciousness* by Dr. Hilton Hotema, I read about an experiment of Claude

Bernard conducted with birds. He showed that if a bird is placed under a bell-glass of such size that the air contained within will permit the bird to live for three hours, and the bird is removed at the end of the second hour, when it could have survived another hour, and a fresh healthy bird is put in place, the latter will die at once. The second bird was not adjusted to the reduced oxygen. The bird that survived three hours adjusted to the oxygen change slowly. This enabled the first bird to survive longer. The second bird did not have time to adjust, the change was too abrupt.

The point is that bodies adjust to survive. Our human bodies have adjusted to many outside forces and stimuli in order to survive. Think of all we humans adjusted to: radiation from microwaves, wearing glasses, wearing shoes, noise pollution, air pollution, going to school, chlorinated water, violence, violent thoughts, the same temperature all the time in a room, television, music, lack of sleep, doughnuts, lack of exercise, bad eating habits, electric lights, stress, pharmaceutical drugs, driving, synthetic clothes, living in isolation, artificial foods, synthetic vitamins and many more. When our bodies adjust to something, we pay with our health. We pay with our energy and lifespan.

What do we need to do to get more lifespan and more energy now? Be as natural as possible. Stay happy. End pressures. Stop the stress. Sleep outside. Sometimes get cold and wet outside and shiver. Go on a camping trip. We can change what we eat. We can go on raw food. This is doable.

If cooked food isn't the ideal nutritional source for our bodies, how did we get to a diet of 90 - 95% cooked food? Our great, great, great, great, great, great grandfather was a raw fooder, 2000-5000 years ago. I imagine, one day there was a big fire in the woods, all the tubers, plants, and seeds were burned. There was no food. The family was hungry, so he went into the burnt woods and he found a piece of cooked deer there, and he thought to himself, "Eating this is foreign, but it's better than starving." The cooked meat was brought home and consumed. Everyone agreed it was better to change their diet than to starve. Their bodies, reacting to this foreign substance, had one of two choices, to reject the cooked food and die of starvation, or to adjust to the cooked food and live. The bodies adjusted.

How does the body adjust to cooked food? The body creates mucus and uses this mucus as a filter. All the surfaces of the digestive tract that are designed to absorb the nutrients from the food become covered with mucus film that protects blood from toxins. The mucus film begins at the tongue and continues all the way through the intestines. Many people can see this mucus on their tongue. People who have a thick mucus coating on their intestines usually have white tongues as if they just ate sour cream. The body creates a little mucus, to begin with, to filter out the toxins from the cooked food. The more cooked food we consume, the more mucus the body produces as protection. The more harmful the food substances are to the body, the more this mucous film builds up. As the years go by it becomes thicker and harder.

Our body initially creates mucus when we eat our first cooked food as a baby. The next time we eat cooked food the toxins in the food do not penetrate the body completely because of the mucus protection. You may ask: what is the mucus made of? The human body, brilliant as always, creates the mucus from the cooked food itself! This mucus covers our entire digestive tract, to prevent us from absorbing the toxins in cooked food that would make the body sick.

We are afraid of e-coli, salmonella or other bacteria, so we cook, pasteurize and irradiate everything. Food is now highly processed and prepackaged. We eat a lot of cooked food and, therefore, our body creates a lot of mucus.

Naturopaths call this mucus in the intestine by the name of mucoid plaque. Mucoid plaque looks like a green, rubbery hose about twenty-five yards long. Because of the mucoid plaque, our nutrient assimilation becomes low. The mucoid plaque protects us from absorbing toxins, but at the same time we cannot absorb nutrients. The more mucus we have, the fewer nutrients we can receive. After a number of years of eating cooked food, we develop severe nutritional deficiencies, become hungry and malnourished.

We become hungrier and hungrier. We come to the point, like I did eight years ago, that when I was leaving the table, I was already hungry again. We're constantly hungry because our body is desperate for nutrients. Our cells are crying for all the 120 minerals we need. They are asking for sodium and for magnesium, and for copper and zinc. Oh please, I want some potassium! We're constantly hungry for something, but when we eat, only a small percent can be assimilated.

When we go on raw food and if we stay on raw food, this mucoid plaque can be dissolved. When the time is right, the body will dissolve it. The more we eat raw food, the more plaque gets dissolved. If we go 100% raw, it goes away completely and our assimilation goes up. When we decide to go 100% raw, we don't need to send a telegram to all our organs announcing the change. Our body hears the message and begins to change right away and begins to celebrate. It

says, "Hey! He/she decided to go raw. Did you hear that?
He/she's going 100% raw!"

The following table shows how the amount of cooked
food we eat in our diet relates to the amount of food that is
assimilated in our body. This table is my hypothesis, it is the
result of an extensive reading, together with a study of cases
of many people on a raw food diet. Sadly, I don't have funds
to conduct scientific research and prove my theory.

Percentage Cooked Food to Raw Food
Consumed & Percentage Nutrition Assimilated

% of raw food	% cooked food	% assimilation
5	95	.03
10	90	.06
25	75	.1
50	50	.3
75	25	1.0
99	1	3.0
100	0	30.0

I'd like to explain this table by way of an illustration.
We'll call the main character Jim, age between 40 and 50. Jim
eats very little raw food. He is always hungry because he is
not getting enough nutrients. He has a big belly because he
eats a lot to try to fill the hunger in his body. He has a weak
back because of the big belly, and he's always tired. Jim consumes a diet that is 5% raw. Anyone who makes sandwiches
or buys hamburgers is eating about 5% raw because the
tomatoes and lettuce make up the 5%. At this point Jim's
body is assimilating approximately .03% of the nutrition in

the food. Let's say Jim got really, really sick. He goes to a health store and learns that he might feel better if he eats a vegetarian diet. He adds a lot of fresh food to his diet and cuts out the meat. He is now consuming 25% raw food and 75% cooked food. His assimilation increased three times to .1% or 1/10%. He's starting to feel better and he has a little more energy. He hangs out with his new friends who are also vegetarians. One of them invites him to a raw food potluck. Jim is so impressed with the dishes and the presentation that he increases his raw food intake to 50%. He is now assimilating .3% or 3/10%. As far as assimilation goes, this is a lot. This is actually 10 times more than he had before. He sees the difference. He begins to feel good. Jim begins to come to every weekly potluck and he increases his raw food intake to 75% while the cooked food intake is reduced to 25%. He is now assimilating 1%. 1% is a lot, a good number, 30 times more than he used to have. He begins to look like an interesting man. Jim used to think that no woman would ever look at him, because he was getting old and aching. Now he looks healthy, he's looking younger and his color is coming back.

Jim begins to read a lot of books on raw food eating and he even begins to teach his own raw food class. He is now consuming 99% raw food and 1% cooked food. And he is assimilating about 3%. Jim is so healthy now that he looks 10 years younger. He has a lot of friends and he is very social. Everyone loves him. We check in with Jim several years later. He has read many raw food books and has gone to every possible retreat and class offered on raw food. One morning he wakes up and hears his inner voice telling him to give up cooked food all together and to go 100% on raw food. He makes that choice. Within two or three months of consuming only raw foods, his assimilation becomes 30%. His assimilation has increased from 3.0% to 30% in just two to three months. Why did changing his diet from 99% raw food to 100% raw food make such a difference in his assimilation rate? The 1% is significant because his body's defense against cooked food is now taken away. He now begins to eat only once a day, a small bowl of salad, that's it. He only needs one small bowl because he is assimilating 30%. Remember when Jim was eating 95% cooked food and ate a lot to feed his starving body? At that point he was only assimilating .03%. Now on a 100% raw food diet, Jim is assimilating 30% nutrition. This is why he only needs a small amount of food to satisfy him. That's enough for this man. That's how much I eat. That's how much my husband eats. That's how much my children eat.

When my son Sergei, who is 16, goes snowboarding, he leaves at 6:30 a.m. and comes home at 7:00 p.m. He takes with him two organic oranges to eat on the shuttle bus. He eats one on the way up to the snow and one on the way back home. That's enough because he assimilates 30%.

Sergei says that his snowboarding friends go several times to their lunch bags to drink hot chocolate and eat sandwiches because they get so hungry. They get hungry and have energy crashes and have to go eat. Meanwhile, Sergei is snowboarding all day and he's never tired, and all this on two oranges. The secret is that he is assimilating 30% while they are assimilating only between .03 and .1%. Going back to Jim as an example, why did the final 1% shift from eating 99% to 100% raw food make such a difference in the assimilation rate? I gleaned the answer to this from the Alcoholics Anonymous (AA) literature.

Alcoholics are encouraged at AA meetings to get 100% sober. If they return to the meeting and say they are 99% sober, because they drink only one shot of vodka every other day, they will be told that they are not sober. AA members have noticed a long time ago that quitting 99% doesn't ever work. If someone wants to quit drinking he/she needs to go "cold turkey" or 100%. This last 1%, no matter how small it is, will keep a body adjusted to being a drinker.

We can use this analogy for cooked food too. For example, Andrew has been consuming cooked rice since childhood, his body has adjusted biochemically and psychologically to this consumption. One day Andrew became aware that white rice is not healthy for him. He decided to stop eating rice. As a result Andrew's body has developed strong craving for cooked rice. Cravings are biochemical and emotional expectations of the body. His body has been adjusted to receive carbohydrates from cooked rice. Andrew started to consume carbohydrates from raw corn, sprouted grains and carrots. After two months Andrew's body readjusted and his rice cravings stopped. If Andrew would continue to eat rice even in tiny quantities, his body readjustment would never be completed and Andrew would continue to experience cravings for rice.

Secondly, when we eat, say, a baked potato is there a mark on the potato that says this is 1%, this is 10%? Do we always know when to stop? Also, our parents taught us that we have to finish our food because there are children in China that are starving to death. So we cannot just throw food away, we have to finish it, even if it's more than 1%.

And so, when we allow 1%, we leave the door open to indulge when we feel like it. When we are depressed or hungry or angry or tired that's when we overeat. That's when we indulge in eating cooked food, drinking alcohol, smoking or taking drugs. Giving up the last 1% of cooked food in the diet is closing the door on cooked food all together. When we close the door on cooked food we close the door on temptation.

When our family went on raw food 100% eight years ago, our dear friend Judy also went on raw food. But she went on raw food only 95%. I suffered for two months during my body's adjustment of going completely off cooked food and eating only raw food. After two months, I was no longer attracted to cooked food. I had lost my appetite for cooked food. I stopped paying attention to restaurants or to the smells of food or coffee. I have lived for three years in Ashland, Oregon and I don't even know the name of one restaurant. I know three health food stores and I know a juice bar. I don't pay attention to anything else. Cooked food looks like plastic to me, inedible. That's how I feel. I am not tempted to eat cooked food because it no longer looks like food to me.

My friend, Judy, however, is still suffering. She stays on raw food for weeks at a time, and then company will come to visit and she'll eat cooked food again. She reports, "I stayed for two weeks on 95% raw food diet and then my aunt came to visit and she made a beautiful baked cake and I had to try it. Then I started to eat more cooked food. I failed. I fell back." She has also said, "I was doing very well until Thanksgiving, and then I decided I would take a break until after Thanksgiving. It took me until the second week in February to reclaim my 95% raw food diet." By keeping the door to cooked food open, even 1%, my dear friend Judy is prolonging her suffering.

On 99% we are still addicted and we allow ourselves what

we want, when we want it. I have met many people who have achieved 99% raw food only to return to completely cooked food months later. This tiny 1% will inevitably lead us back to cooked food. What I'm trying to say is that going cold turkey is much easier. Yes, you might have to suffer through two months because every temptation will create suffering. But after two months, life is easier.

Take all temptations (cooked food, processed food, take out menus) out of your house and don't go out to the restaurant, birthday parties and cooked food potlucks for at least two months. Create a temptation free zone. The easier way to become 100% raw is to make the change consciously. Do not become a raw fooder until you feel completely ready.

When you understand that cooked food is addictive, you want to stay on 100% raw food. Becoming a raw fooder without the necessary support is hard. I know some people who understand raw food is good, and they became raw fooders and they stayed as long as six months, but at certain times they became hungry, or lonely, or depressed, or tired and they returned to what is familiar to them, cooked food.

CHAPTER FOUR

Bacteria, My Favorite Animal In The World

I want to share with you my amusement and appreciation for bacteria. Maybe your respect for it will grow after reading this chapter. Bacteria is the world's greatest recycler. Please think about it: by transforming all dead organic matter into the soil, bacteria recycle useless garbage into the original source of all elements. Bacteria is unique, it is tiny and huge at the same time. Smaller than any living cell, bacteria can instantly increase its power by multiplying into zillions more. Bacteria is God's brilliant invention and gift to us all! We are constantly trying to destroy as many bacteria as possible because we don't understand its purpose on Earth. Let us imagine life without bacteria. There would be rocks but no soil in which to grow food. All dead trees, animals, birds, insects, snakes, human bodies or any organic matter would be piled into huge mountains. What a clutter that would be!

In a natural setting, bacteria in the rotting cycle does not cause an odor. Hard to believe? In the forest nobody rakes the leaves, nobody buries the animals, everything is just left in the open. The droppings of animals and birds are left where they've fallen. You would think the forest would smell really bad. So, let me ask you, the last time you were in the forest, did it smell bad? I bet your answer is "no." In fact, when we go to the forest, we breathe in and say, "Ah, it smells so good!" If bacteria acting on organic matter doesn't smell in the natural habitat of the forest, then why do we associate rotting with odor? Why, in the civilized world, does bacteria begin to smell bad? This is because bacteria has a hard time recycling what we create. To test this statement, you can do your own experiment. Put raw fruits and vegetables into your compost. You will notice that they will rot and disintegrate without a bad odor. Now, add to your compost some cooked food such as cooked noodles, chicken soup or mashed potatoes. After a few days, you will notice an odor emanating from your compost. The smell will be so bad that your neighbors might call the police. You will not be able to tolerate it. You will have to put dirt on top, because of the unbearable smell. The smell is coming from bacteria trying to break up cooked food.

Another interesting fact is that bacteria will never touch anything that is still alive. Gigantic redwood trees are 1,000 to 2,000 years old, yet they remain free of bacteria. Their roots are always in the soil, yet bacteria does not touch them. As soon as the tree dies, however, the bacteria moves in to return the tree back to the soil. Bacteria can tell what is living and what is dead and it is only interested in dead matter.

Looking at nature as an example, we see that moss, mistletoe and lichens don't live on strong healthy trees. In an organic garden, if the soil is balanced, the slugs stay out. The worms don't eat healthy tomatoes. Similarly, bacteria and parasites don't live off of healthy flesh. We, as humans, have fallen away from being balanced inside by eating cooked food.

Can bacteria cause disease in humans? Yes and no. Yes, if a human body is filled with toxic waste. No, if a body is clean inside. Bacteria is not interested in our muscles, heart, eyes or brain but only in recycling toxins in our body. The more waste and toxic matter we accumulate in the body the more we attract bacteria. That is why people who eat mostly cooked food get infections so easily. If you are afraid of infectious disease, the best thing you can do is keep your insides clean. Eating raw food is a good way to do this.

The same applies to any parasites. If we keep our body clean, healthy and pure, parasites cannot live off it and even mosquitoes won't bite us. Once my family went to hike in Minnesota where the mosquito is the state bird. In the Boundary Waters Wilderness the forest rangers had to wear mosquito nets around their heads, and we didn't even suffer one bite. There were five of us, all on 100% raw food. For all five nights we didn't even put up tents. We were not bitten. We think we heard those mosquitoes talking to each other and saying, "These are strange people! They are alkaline! Yuck!"

All parasites leave a human body, when it becomes clean. Here is an example to illustrate this point. Just after we began raw foods, we read a book about the parasites humans carry around in their bodies. We were so frightened by the thought of these parasites, that we decided to do a family parasite cleanse. For ten days we ate special tablets to cleanse

the body of parasites. Two months later we took a blood test
and saw that the parasites were back. The tablet cleanse only
kept us clean for two months. One and a half years later, after
being on a 100% raw food diet the entire time, we did the
same blood test. Our blood was pristine! There were no parasites at all! Our blood consisted of only blood cells; red blood
cells, and white blood cells. That's all that was there. There
was no bacteria. We were clean.

When we look at a person's blood who eats cooked
food, we can usually see lots of bacteria floating in between
the blood cells. Once I invited a specialist, who performs
Dark Field Live Blood Analysis, to my class to demonstrate
live blood cell analysis. He took blood samples from three
volunteers. One of the volunteers was a young man of 19. His
blood was so penetrated with parasites and bacteria
that he became embarrassed!

He said, "But I take a shower every day." I said, "Don't be
embarrassed, the parasites and bacteria in your blood have
nothing to do with how many showers you take. Tell us about
your lifestyle." He said, "Oh, I'm getting better." We said, "Just
relax, and tell us, what do you eat? What are your habits?
How have you been living the last 19 years of your life?"
He said, "I've been taking drugs, I drink beer, I was diagnosed
with AIDS, I was diagnosed with testicle cancer, I was smoking marijuana, I was eating junk food (pizza was my favorite
food), and I never liked salads."

We could see this in his blood. No matter how much we
wash ourselves outside, inside we can be very infected.
Bacteria knows right away where the toxins are. Bacteria
is dedicated to its work. Without any pain (thank God it's
small!), bacteria penetrates inside the human body and into

the cells, multiplies and begins to work. Bacteria is helping our body get rid of toxins.

What I know for sure is that people who eat raw foods don't have parasites or harmful bacteria. People who have been tested and told by doctors that they have parasites have been able to get rid of these parasites by eating a 100% raw food diet. Doctors are surprised when parasites disappear because usually it is hard to get rid of them (parasites exist in all kinds of shapes and different stages, and if you kill one stage, then another stage will continue to develop). When we begin to eat raw food, our body cleanses itself of toxins. There is nothing left for the parasites to eat, so they leave.

CHAPTER FIVE

Detoxification as Healing

When we first eat cooked food, as a baby, the cooked food creates the first mucus in the body. Some of the mucus is used to create a film along the digestive tract while the excess mucus is stored in the most convenient place, the lungs. Mucus is not supposed to stay in lungs permanently, so the lungs have a mechanism, similar to peristalsis, to move the mucus out. It looks like millions of little fingers on the surface of the lungs that work as a moving belt to clear mucus out the lungs. This mechanism takes pieces of mucus out of the lungs and moves them to the nose - then we see that the baby has a runny nose. When we feed our baby mucus-forming food, the baby will have a runny nose all the time as the body is trying to move the mucus out. That would be perfectly okay from nature's point of view: all the excess of mucus would get evacuated through the baby's nose and the lungs would stay clear. But, what do we do when we see a runny nose in our baby? The typical response is, "Wow! My baby has a runny nose. The skin is already irritated. He has a rash around his poor little nose. I need to help my baby. I'll take him to the doctor." The doctor prescribes nose drops. We feel better because we've done what we can to help our baby.

I want to argue that the nose drops are not necessary. The baby is not nose drop deficient. The drops are toxic. They are so toxic, that the body stops moving the mucus out of the lungs and begins to concentrate on how to get rid of the toxins from the nose drops. So, the body stops the cleaning process, the runny nose stops and the mucus goes back into the lungs. We look at our baby and say, "Yes, those nose drops worked. My baby is well." We don't realize that the nose stopped running because the body concentrated energy on evacuating the toxic drops. And that the red runny nose is not as dangerous as the lungs filled with mucus plus the body weakend by the toxic nose drops. Meanwhile, the mucus layer gets thicker. It takes a lot of energy for the body to clear mucus out of the lungs. When the body has built up enough energy, it will begin to clear the mucus again.

So, about three months later, the baby will start to have a runny nose again. What do we do? We think, "The runny nose is back, I'd better call the doctor." We take the baby to the doctor who tells us that we need stronger nose drops this time because there is more mucus now, and this mucus is more concentrated, so it makes the tonsils swollen. Mucus also creates a hoarse voice, because it travels through the trachea, covering the vocal chords.

The new, stronger medicine is so toxic, that the body stops detoxing in order to focus on clearing out the medicine. It might take another several months for the baby's body to build enough energy to create another effort to detox.

Think for a minute, when in your life do you usually have more energy than average? You have more energy when you go on vacation, or on the weekend if you are relaxing. When do you usually get sick? Have you ever said, "It never fails, I have some time off and I get sick." When your body receives extra energy, it rushes to use it before it is used for something else. Your body uses this energy to detox. That is why we tend to get sick when we have "down" time.

To hasten the removal of toxins the body creates fever. Fever is not just a high temperature of the body, but is a complex process that requires time and energy. In order to create a fever, the body has to work hard. The heart has to pump 20 to 30 heartbeats faster per minute than usual. All the hormonal glands have to do extra work. That is why we feel tired. To conserve the energy used to digest food, the body creates a no-appetite condition. The tongue is coated with a thick layer of mucus so we cannot feel the taste; the nose is stuffed so we cannot be tempted by the smell of the food; the tonsils are swollen so it is hard to swallow. What happens when the body has a fever? The body goes into a sweat so that the mucus can come out through the pores. Do you remember that particular sticky and smelly sweat that happens during high fever? The mucus becomes more lique-fied and we get very runny noses.

A common response to fever is to take an aspirin. Why do we do that? We are not aspirin deficient. Aspirin is largely sulfur and sulfur is bad for us. Our body doesn't expect that kind of cruelty from us. Sulfur is so toxic that the body sim-ply doesn't have enough energy to continue evacuation of mucus. The important process of healing stops. All the body is concerned with now is aspirin in the blood. A priority is to get rid of it as soon as possible. To do so the body is compelled to work so hard and gets so weak that it cannot even continue to maintain a normal body temperature. Our temperature then falls below normal. We have to stay in bed because we feel weak. The body's response to aspirin makes us feel so weak, not the fever.

To add insult to injury, when we are feeling weak, we eat heavy food, like chicken soup. We have no appetite. Our body is saying, "Don't eat!" And yet, we think we need to eat chicken soup so that we will "have energy." I used to do that to my children. I used to say, "Have some chicken soup, you need energy," or I'd feed them something else high in calories. In response to eating in this "Don't eat" stage, if the body still has a little bit of energy left, it will create a throw-up situation. It will say, "No, no not this, I need all of my energy for healing." If we eat when the body is in the "Don't eat" stage, the blood has to go into the stomach to process the chicken soup thereby taking the energy away from the detox. Eating takes a lot of energy and can make us feel even weaker. This is how not cooperating with our body can affect us.

Recovering from taking medication takes energy. After one illness, we may not get sick for a long time. That is because there is no energy in the body for detox. The body has to store up energy before it can begin a healing event again. That is why most adults never have such a high fever as they did in their childhood.

Meanwhile, the mucus in the lungs builds up. The fresh mucus layer is clear. The older mucus is green, or dark orange, brown or yellow. To get rid of this heavy mucus build up, the body might create pneumonia. The body is making a heroic effort to clear itself of mucus. This takes even more energy than fever and we feel very tired. There is a gasping and raspy sound when we breathe. When we have pneumonia, we use penicillin. This stops the mucus evacuation and further weakens the body.

For many years the body will have no more detox, except a little "cold" now and then, which is a very weak attempt by the body to detox. The body will continue to store the excess mucus in the lungs until there is about one-third lung space left, and at this point the lungs say, "I cannot take any more. I need this one-third to continue breathing, to continue living. I cannot live on less oxygen than that." There is a little extra storage in the sinuses and in the forehead. The mucus moves to these areas. Next, the body begins to use a layer under the skin to store the mucus. When we have mucus and toxins stored in a layer under our skin, first we develop goose bumps or rough skin that is not very silky. Then when we walk just a little bit we begin to sweat a little, and mucus begins to pour through our skin pores. This mucus is acidic; it irritates the skin. If you will pour lots of lemon juice on your skin and rub it in, you will feel itchiness. When this acid mucus comes through, our skin feels itchy. We call it an allergy. Why does an allergy happen? Why does it exist? We have lots of toxins in the body. People say, "It happens when I eat citrus." Citrus only dissolves this toxin, and helps move it through the skin faster. This is actually good for us. This really means we have an enormous amount of toxins.

Sometimes, we accumulate so much mucus in our body that we develop a condition of labored breathing with wheezing that is called asthma. We cannot breathe. We don't have enough oxygen. We don't have enough space to breath we're so filled with mucus. The mucus stored in the forehead, very close to the brain, causes headaches, and potentially brain tumors. That space was not meant to be permanently filled up with mucus.

I'll give you a simple way to tell if you have mucus in your lungs. Run around the block. If you have mucus coming out of your nose, then you do. If you can run two times around the block, and you have no mucus running out of your nose, you have clean lungs. If you can breathe through your nose when you're running, you don't have any mucus. Have you ever noticed that professional runners have to spit up phlegm when they are in a race? They eat their cooked vegan or vegetarian diet with lots of high calorie meals like rice and baked potatoes which are mucus forming foods. When raw fooders run, they don't have any mucus. I know many raw fooders who run, and they don't have any problem with mucus, they don't need to spit, and they can breathe through their noses. They have enough oxygen to run and talk. Their lungs are clean.

Our body was meant to be cleaned by running. We are animals that are at least supposed to walk. That is why we have a limited amount of storage for the mucus. We were built to move. We have this mechanism, when we're moving and shaking, the lungs begin to pump and push the mucus out. But if we don't run or rarely walk, how do we expect our body to take out the mucus? Instead of helping our body to rid itself of mucus, we short circuit its effort and take an aspirin.

The body has to be very strong to create a fever. When we are able to create a really good fever, we should celebrate! Be very happy. The body is dedicated for you to be very healthy. When you have a fever, help your body by not eating food. You probably won't want to eat when you have a fever anyway. When I was little and had a fever, I never wanted to eat, and my mother was always trying to feed me. She would give me hot milk. Milk, with butter on the top. And all kinds of yucky stuff, but I never wanted to eat it. If you want to help, you can do body wraps, or alternate cold and hot showers, take a bath. Do what your body wants. Your body is clear about what it wants. You either want the covers off or on. But usually when I took my blanket off, my mother would say, "Oh no, no, no, keep that on. Don't get cold." My mother was doing what she thought was best for me. Now we know that the best we can do is to listen to our bodies. All of us have toxins in our body. Detoxing is our body's effort to clear out these toxins. Detoxing is unavoidable in order to become healthy. What are the major symptoms of detoxification? Before I tell you this, I want to share with you a story.

When I worked at the Creative Health Institute (CHI), guests would come for two to six weeks to learn how to eat raw food. First they were put on a two day juice fast, and then they were fed wheat grass, sprouts and raw food. Every day the guests met with the staff to assess and discuss the symptoms of detox or healing events. Guests would report symptoms of rash, headache, diarrhea, cold sores and weakness. There was usually one guest in every group who had no symptoms at all. Rather than being good news, the staff knew that having no symptoms of detox was a warning sign. It meant that the guest's body had no energy left to create a healing condition. This is why I want you to celebrate the symptoms of healing events. When you go on raw foods, you immediately give lots of energy back to your body. You are supposed to have a detox. If you don't have it, it could be the sign of some problem. So, if any of you decide to go on raw food, expect to have a healing event. Even if you have detox symptoms on an inconvenient day, when you have a presentation or are at a conference, it doesn't matter, be grateful. If you have detoxing signs, you need to celebrate! Feel happy! Rejoice!

What are the most common symptoms of detox? About 75% of people, when they go on raw foods, experience cold sores in the mouth. Cold sores happen because the saliva becomes very acidic, irritates the gums and creates a cold sore. Cold sores are annoying, painful and irritating. There is nothing you can do. You cannot wash or rinse or put on any oil. You have to wait until your saliva changes. When you first go on raw food, your body is going to start cleaning you out by throwing all accumulated waste into the blood. This creates a temporary acidic condition. That's why when we are fasting, we smell bad. When we fast or change our diet radically, we smell like ammonia.

Another type of detoxing symptom is weakness. Most people experience a few hours of weakness in the first week. Once in a while, we will get so suddenly weak we cannot even move our finger. Then just as suddenly, it goes away and we have more energy than we did before. The weakness is felt when the body takes time and energy to clean certain organs. Imagine a scanning machine looking through the whole body. All of a sudden it finds an organ that needs fixing. The scanning machine sends a message out to the body's energy center. It says, "Oops, there's something in here. I need to spend some time in here, and I need to spend some extra energy." That's how the body works.

Another symptom is headaches. If you have eaten a lot of white sugar in your life or had coffee or if you've taken painkillers, you will probably experience headaches. These headaches usually won't last for more than two or three days, but they may seem unbearable. To help yourself feel better, lie down and rest, take a bath, sleep or give yourself an enema. Ask you body, "What do you need?" and listen.

Rashes are another common symptom. About 90% of people experience a rash one to three times. Our body divides all the toxins into certain groups. One group is eliminated through the ears. Another is easier to eliminate through the nose. Some toxins have to be eliminated through the skin in the sweat. Whenever the toxin is being released through the skin, you will experience some kind of a rash. The more acidic the sweat is, the more unbearable the rash will be. What do you do when you have a rash? Take a hot bath and sweat. Go to the sauna. If you go to the sauna, remember you need to wash the toxic sweat off. I go to the sauna often, because where I live there is a sauna. I have watched people get into the sauna. Their body works to sweat out all the toxins and then they go in the open, cold air, sit down and dry off. The body then reabsorbs all those toxins back! When our pores are open, our body is like a sponge, absorbing everything back. We need to wash off the sweat and the toxins. Cold water is best as the pores will squeeze extra toxins out as they close.

The next symptom is diarrhea. Some people have diarrhea, which is great. I once prayed for diarrhea and I didn't get it. Once my friend didn't pray for it, and he had it for six months on and off. He couldn't go to the movies because he was afraid to go further than 100 feet from the house. I wanted diarrhea because I had a prolapsed colon, and I had been told that diarrhea would straighten my colon. Diarrhea is not bad and is not caused by bacteria. Diarrhea is caused by the body trying to clean itself.

When you experience detox symptoms, the first thing to do is to call somebody in the raw food community who will understand and talk with you. You can call another raw fooder and say, "I'm calling you because I'm dying! I am having such a terrible headache, everything is shaking, and I have weakness." And your friend, understanding the detox process, will say, "Congratulations, your body is working!" Why reach out to other raw fooders? It is important because, no matter how much I explain, when the actual detox happens you will panic. Everybody does. This is why it is very important to call someone who can reaffirm your choice for health and that can reassure you that you are all right. Someone to tell you everything is okay and that what you are feeling is normal.

If you are experiencing a healing event, you may consider fasting on water or juice for 24-36 hours. Fasting will speed up the process of detoxification. Read books on fasting before you plan to do so. If you want to fast for a longer period, going to a fasting clinic would be your safest choice.

CHAPTER SIX

The Family Fast

Fasting is a privilege. Fasting is joy. When is a good time to fast? You will know it is time to fast when everything becomes untasty. You will eat your favorite food and it just won't taste good. That is the sign that your body is ordering you to fast.

I fasted on water many times from one day to twenty-one days. Sometimes I do a several day juice fast. Our family of four enjoys fasting together. Often we fast together one or two days while driving long distances to our workshops. That makes our trips easier and we don't get tired. As a family we have done several seven day juice fasts and many one or two day water fasts.

In February of this year our family completed a fourteen day water fast. It brought our family so close together! Every day we gathered at home to share all the things that were happening with our bodies. We were all going through the same experience together. We asked each other: "Do you experience this? Do you experience that? You do? Oh good." On the third day, all of us experienced physical weakness.

Valya was answering the phone while I was gone for two hours. My phone is always ringing. Valya had to hold her arm up to answer the phone. Her arm hurt for the rest of the day just from holding the phone. Sergei was on the mountain snowboarding that day. An hour after he arrived, he called home, "Can you come and get me, I can't even pull my snowboard in the snow." We decided that our weakness happened because our bodies were switching from feeding on actual food, feeding on bodily internal reserves. On the fourth day we all experienced energy. Sergei snowboarded all day. Sergei was so excited to tell his friends that he was on his third day of a water fast. His friends didn't believe him. One boy said Sergei was just making it up, and that he didn't look like he hadn't eaten. On the evening of our fifth day we hugged together as a family. "Guys, this is our fifth day!" We asked one another, "Are we going to fast another week and a half as planned? Gosh, another week and a half seems so long." Then we started to notice how much free time we had. During the day we saved a lot of time that we normally would have spent shopping, preparing and eating. Instead of food, for those two weeks, we decided we were going to go to the sauna, as a family, at lunchtime every single day. Because we were missing the nice smells of the food, we bought lemon tincture and put it in the sauna and smelled lemon. We had lots of energy. We woke up right as the sun came up and went to bed around midnight. We liked to observe each other's figures, and see what was different and how we were all getting into shape. We went swimming. It was just a wonderful experience! Sergei said, "I never knew I was so hooked on the ritual of eating."

Toward the end of the fast, Sergei called a friend and said,

"Do you want my skateboard? Come and get it! I decided I'm not going to skateboard anymore. It's just a waste of time. I'm going to read more now." After finishing the fast, Sergei doubled his college classes. He doubled his music lessons. He wrote an article for a magazine. He seemed to mature during the fasting process. Now he is teaching a raw food class in our town. After the fast, he became a little wizard. It was a beautiful experience to observe. Valya seemed to become more confident in herself after this fast, she was constantly in a very happy, joyous mood.

Towards the end of the fast, we began to experience days when some of us during different times would experience weakness. That's when the body needed some energy for healing. Then we would lie down and rest. When the energy returned we knew that the certain part of healing was complete. We had lots of energy. Oh, precious energy!

On the thirteenth night of the fast, I had a dream. In the dream I was sitting on a tricycle. I was three years old and my father was spraying the garden with DDT. I got off my bike and walked behind my dad towards the box with poison and put my hands in this white powder. It smelled so bad . . . I woke up, and I had a DDT taste in my mouth. I went to the bathroom and started to wash my mouth, but the chemical taste wouldn't wash out. It came together with the actual memory from my childhood, when my father was spraying the garden with DDT, with me sitting on the tricycle. I also remembered that there was no asphalt for the street yet, I had to ride my tricycle on just boards. It is interesting to me that I remembered this episode with DDT spraying so vividly. I know my body was now clearing out the poison that had been in my body since I was three.

In the end of the fast we wondered how should we break it? We have several fasting books and they each suggest a different way to break the fast. One tells us to break our fast with juice, another says, wheat grass, yet another says oranges, and another says peeled tomatoes. We decided to meditate as a family and listen to our bodies to see what they wanted. Then we heard the answer, just in time, very clearly. We were going to have grated organic Fuji apples, several chunks of organic pineapple and several pieces of prunes. Then we were going to stay on juices for three days.

The kids arrived home from college by bus at 5:20 p.m. and Igor and I had a beautiful table with flowers in the middle, and everybody had a platter with a pile of grated apple, chunks of pineapple, and soaked prunes, and the prune water in the middle. I made a poster "Congratulations Boutenko Family on Successfully Finishing Our 14 Day Water Fast!" When the kids came in, and they hadn't eaten for two weeks, and they saw this beautiful table with beautiful plates, and the food smells. Wow!!!

We sat as a family and held hands together. "Should we really eat?" Sergei said. "I wish we could wait another day!" Valya said. Then we started to eat. Oh, it was so good! None of us could finish even half a plate. We felt so full. Our stomachs had shrunk. Oh, I wish I could eat more! We had to leave it for later. A couple hours later we finished everything, then we stood for a long time together, hugging and feeling how we were so glad we did it. Thank you, all of you! We were just feeling such a tremendous thankfulness, and togetherness, and joy.

During the fast, Valya was taking jazz lessons where they had really vigorous exercises. After she went twice during the fast, she said, "You know Mom, I don't know if I can go a third time and really do everything, because I felt sometimes I couldn't really hold my hands up for a long time. I wanted to sit down and just rest." When the teacher would turn away, Valya would put her hands down, and when the teacher turned back, she'd put them back up.

I mixed a special drink for Valya. Half Thai coconut water and half distilled water in a cup had enough glucose to give her a little bit of energy. So, for the children in the last few days, if they needed to go to an exercise class, I gave them one cup of this water mixed with coconut water, and it worked. Igor and I didn't take any coconut water, but Valya and Sergei did.

Fasting as a family was a beautiful experience. I encouraged our kids to take notes and they did. Now Sergei says he would like to fast one or two times per year again as a family and write a book called *Family Fasting*. Both kids did lose almost 20 pounds each, and they did look thin, but they gained back 10 pounds within the first three days of juicing. It was amazing. We all enjoyed our newest experience in fasting. We cannot wait until the next time we fast as a family again.

PART TWO

How to
Stay Raw

CHAPTER SEVEN

Why Twelve Steps?

I would like to ask you a question: Is food your number one pleasure? Before rushing to say no, think about how we celebrate special dates. Do we fast on our birthdays, our wedding day or holidays? Do we go for a walk to celebrate these occasions or do we make fancy and abundant feasts? When we attend an anniversary party, do we expect to be nicely fed? How would we feel about the party if no food was offered?

Food is synonymous with celebration in our culture. For holiday dinners we plan delicious meals and buy the most mouth-watering items to eat. We even have special celebration dishes such as tortes, chocolate truffles, fancy cakes, candy and appetizers that we associate with each holiday. We look forward to eating as part of the holiday celebration!

How do you feel after a holiday dinner? Can you describe honestly how your body feels the next morning? Do you feel sleepy, tired or wrung out? Do you need coffee? Have you noticed that your body tends to feel this way after big holiday meals? Even if we answer yes, does this uncomfortable feeling stop us from planning our next holiday meal?

If we ate just for nutrition, would we eat potato chips or drink coffee or beer? When we go to the deli section and admire the fancy dishes in the deli case, are we admiring the nutritional quality of the food or the taste potential and pleasure that the food offers? Most of us would probably answer pleasure. When we recognize that food is the number one pleasure for the majority of us, we can then become aware of the fact that we consume food not for its nutritional value, but for pleasure.

When we want our food to bring us pleasure first and nutrition second, then nutritional value is sacrificed for the taste. Because of this, we end up with food that has very stimulating taste and very little nutritional value. These are the two main characteristics of cooked food. Raw food, however, can give us both nutritional value and pleasure.

I started to teach classes about raw foods eight years ago. As soon as I lost my first 30 pounds, I gathered neighbors and friends in my house and started to tell them about the health benefits I had experienced by eating only raw foods. They got really excited and decided to become raw too. However, none of them lasted on raw food even through the next morning's breakfast. I met some of my students a couple days later at the store and I asked them how was their raw life. One friend said, "I cannot become raw yet. I have to cook for my family." Others tried to avoid me. I decided that I did not do a good job teaching them how to eat raw if they couldn't stay on it. I decided to study more. I visited different alternative healing centers and read day and night. I started to teach again and this time I put all my talents into the class. I sang, I danced Russian folk dances, I told jokes. I tried everything I could to make enzymes and sprouts interesting.

By the end of the class, everyone got very excited and said, "Oh, I'm not going to eat cooked food ever again in my life. I'm going to eat only raw." But as I learned later, my new students' raw food life didn't last through breakfast either. I met two of my students in the store the next week and they were hiding their muffins behind their back and saying, "Sorry Victoria, we couldn't make it." I knew something was wrong with my teaching and I didn't like it that my friends were hiding from me as if I were the police! I decided to shut my mouth until I found a way I could teach so people would follow. My goal became to meet other raw food teachers and chefs and to learn from them how to teach the raw food lifestyle successfully.

For two and a half years we traveled around the country and visited many alternative healing centers. We came across several places where the raw food lifestyle was taught. People with cancer, diabetes, allergies, asthma and other serious illnesses came to these health centers from all over the world and stayed, usually for two to six weeks, to learn the raw food lifestyle. The staff taught about raw food and explained why is it the best food for humans. Guests were served beautiful raw meals.

At one such place, the CHI, we stayed for nine months. CHI had the ideal conditions for making a raw food diet most effective. Guests of CHI were completely isolated from any stress and temptations and were in a beautiful and homey atmosphere.

Most of the guests at CHI had been diagnosed with a fatal disease such as cancer. In most cases, they made their decision to try raw food as a last resort. Most had already gone through chemotherapy and radiation and their doctors had told them that there was nothing else that could be done to help them.

The guests of CHI were introduced to a 100% raw diet and all 132 guests reported feeling better. They observed their tumors shrinking in a matter of weeks, other symptoms of disease were reduced and they felt good. The guests pledged to stay on raw food as it had helped them to feel better. When families came to visit, they were also supportive of the raw diet lifestyle as they could see a difference in their loved one's health. It was clear to many guests that the raw food diet was enabling them to live longer. We were all very happy for the guests and their healing experiences. As they left, we wished them well.

As a follow up, I asked Don Haughey, owner of CHI, if he had done any research on how many of his guests actually stayed on the raw diet after they went home? He paused for a long moment, sighed and answered, "About 2%. When they go home they don't stay on the diet." I was mystified. "Do they choose to die?" I asked. He didn't answer, a tear came down his cheek. I couldn't find an explanation as to why people were unable to stay on raw food even when they had personally experienced the extraordinary health benefits and were dedicated to the raw lifestyle. This became a real mystery to me and I wanted to solve the puzzle.

As I thought over this puzzle, I continued to teach classes. My students were always excited about going on a raw food diet and I taught them how to prepare delicious raw meals, but still not many of them remained raw. I was becoming tired and discouraged.

Then one day a friend invited me to an AA meeting that was open to the public. As I listened to the talk at the meeting

I could see it all so clearly. Cooked food is an addiction! That is why will power and the best intentions do not keep one on the raw lifestyle. At last I got the puzzle answered. I felt so happy! It was a revelation!

I went to the public library and asked for books on addictions. The librarian showed me many shelves full of books. I asked, "How many books can I check out?" The answer was, "38 books." So, I checked out 38 books on all kinds of addictions, from drugs and alcohol to overspending and overeating. I read all 38 books and returned for more until I'd read them all. The librarian was sure I had a BIG problem.

Next, I made a trip to the biggest bookstore in our town. I spent the whole day there reading and brought more books home. One book was written by two medical professors and had a universal questionnaire on addiction to any chemical substance. If a person answered "yes" on more than three questions from the questionnaire, then that person had an addiction to that particular addictive substance.

As an experiment I made a copy of the questionnaire, whited out "chemical substance" and typed in "cooked food." I gave it to all of my students in three classes and everybody answered "yes" to most of the questions. I thought, "Hallelujah, that's the proof, it's an addiction. Wow! That is so radical!" I felt as if I jumped off the Empire State Building. But the more I gave it a thought, the more it made sense to me.

There are hundreds of thousands of people who want to be raw fooders. They have learned about the health benefits of eating raw foods and sincerely want to change their diets. Some of these people feel compelled to go on a raw food diet by a serious illness. But when these people begin to eat raw

food they discover that to stay on a 100% raw diet is so hard,
almost impossible! Only a few people actually stay 100% raw
longer than a year. Even some of the well-known raw food
teachers admit that they can't stay 100% raw. What seems
easy from the first sight in reality appears to be extremely
hard, because cooked food is addictive.

Open the *AA Big Book* and you will read that only one
person out of maybe a 1, 000 could quit drinking alcohol by
sheer will power alone. You will also read that 12 Step programs have helped hundreds of thousands. I believe that if
the 12 Step program works for people with other addictions,
it can also work for people with cooked food addiction.

I understand now that by teaching only why raw food is
good, I could not help anybody. There is about 1 person out
of 1, 000 that can stay on raw food with will power and without support. I have met two or three people who have been
able to stay on raw food for over one year by using only
willpower. The problem with will power is that in times when
you feel angry, hungry, lonely or depressed you turn to
cooked food for comfort.

That is precisely why I developed *12 Steps to Raw Food*.
In the last year and a half I have taught this program in
Washington, Minnesota, Oregon, Arizona, Maryland,
Colorado and California. At first I was afraid. I didn't know
how people would react. I thought, "It's so radical and it's so
different." But then the majority of students who went
through the 12 Steps to Raw Food program have stayed on a
100% raw diet for several months to over a year and they are
continuing to be raw! It's a very powerful program already
and, as I stated earlier, I keep working on improvements.
The 12 Steps to Raw Food program has more differences

than similarities in comparison with other 12 Step programs.
I believe that cooked food is much more cunning, more
cruel, more subtle and thus much more difficult to overcome.

Cooked food is a legal addiction, easy to acquire and is
advertised everywhere. It's not only accepted, but is encouraged. Ingrained in our culture, cooked food is thought to be
normal, proper and healthy. It doesn't even occur to us that
cooked food could be harmful, so we keep looking for a solution somewhere else until we have looked everywhere and
don't find the right answer. All of us who turned to raw food
had some serious reasons for doing so, either health problems, ethical, spiritual or other reasons. For me, it was the
matter of life and death. I knew I would die if I didn't seek
that truth for myself. All members of my family had very
serious health problems before we went on raw food. We
have described our family story in our book *Raw Family*.

Addiction to cooked food is harder and stronger than any
other addiction. In most of the books on drugs they say the
earlier the drugs or chemical substance are taken, the harder
they are to get off. Think about the first time you ate cooked
food. You were most likely about six months to a year old. Did
you like cooked food when you first took a bite? Probably not.
You don't remember. Let us make an analogy. Think back to
when you first tried coffee. How did it taste? Bitter. Did you
ask yourself, "How can adults drink this?" Coffee is an
acquired taste. We ignored our body's response of "ugh, bitter" and kept trying coffee until we got used to it. We did this
because coffee is a social drink and a symbol of adulthood.
Did you like beer the first time you tried it? What about a first
cigarette? Do you remember your body's reaction? "No, get

that away from me!" When we first try anything that is not healthy, our body always gives us a warning. When you first tried cooked food, you probably cried. Maybe you even had a rash. But your mother thought you were teething. So your mother, with the best intentions, continued to feed you cooked food. Then you got used to it and then you got addicted to it.

However, there is a big problem in calling cooked food an addiction. Addiction has a poor reputation in our society. Addiction is a word we don't like to associate with ourselves. None of us want to say, "I am an addict." We don't like others to look down on us. But the truth is that most of us are addicted to something, be it shopping, accumulating things, watching TV or eating sweets, etc. We call these bad habits. We don't like to call them addictions. When we hear the word "addict" we imagine dirty and depressed people who steal money and hurt women and children.

I want to apologize if I hurt anybody's feelings. It is not my intention to offend you or make you feel uncomfortable. What I have found is so incredible and my intention is to share with you, for the good of all.

CHAPTER EIGHT

Step One

I admit that I have lost control of my addiction to cooked food and my eating is becoming unmanageable.

The first step is the hardest one. This is the time in my classes when some people get up, leave the building and slam the door on their way out. I never hear from them again. I apologize if this is the way you feel. Please don't rush to make up your mind. Let us do a little work.

Cooked Food Dependency Questionnaire

This is a questionnaire to determine addiction to cooked food. Please answer "yes" or "no" to each of the following questions. If you want to answer "sometimes," "maybe" or "rare" then answer "yes." Please be honest.

1. If you are not hungry, but someone offers you your favorite delicious food, do you accept the offer?
2. If you know that it is not good to eat before bedtime, but there is some delicious food on the table, do you eat it?

3. If you are feeling stressed, do you eat more food than usual?
4. Do you continue eating until your stomach feels completely full?
5. Do you eat when you are bored?
6. Do you notice restaurant signs even when you are not hungry?
7. If you are made an offer for a free dinner, do you always accept the offer?
8. At All-You-Can-Eat restaurants, do you usually overeat?
9. Have you ever broken a promise to yourself not to eat before bedtime?
10. Would you spend the last $10 in your pocket on your favorite food?
11. Do you reward yourself with food for accomplishing achievements?
12. Do you eat extra food rather than letting it go to waste?
13. If you know that eating a certain food that you really enjoy will make you feel ill later, do you still eat it?

If you answered "yes" to three or more questions, then you may have a cooked-food dependency.

Sometimes raw fooders answer "yes" to more than three questions. Usually that happens to people who are not staying on 100% raw diet or they have just recently become 100% raw. For one and a half years after becoming a 100% raw fooder, I still viewed food as a comforting element. I was still thinking that food was a sign of love, that love was coming from food, and that food was the place to derive comfort and pleasure. This view of food changed when I reached the one and a half year mark. At this point I began to find other pleasurable things in my life. I no longer looked to food for comfort. If you are a raw fooder and you answered yes on three or more questions on the "Cooked Food Dependency Test," don't worry. You will shift your focus after awhile. For those of you who are on raw foods 99%, you may consider food comforting and pleasurable for the rest of your life. Hanging on to that 1% cooked food in your diet keeps you craving cooked food. It's like someone who quits drinking but consumes one shot of vodka every Saturday. Is this person truly sober?

Have you heard the words "rock bottom?" Maybe you heard that one has to "hit rock bottom" in order to end addiction? Imagine people who have been drinking for many years, ruined their health, lost their families and job, their loved ones begged them to quit, but they couldn't. Then suddenly they hit "rock bottom" and a miracle happened, they became sober for good. Have you ever thought about what happens at "rock bottom" and why exactly that place is so powerful? I used to think that the time when one hits "rock bottom" depends on the depth of despair and closeness to death. Do you also think so? Then I have good news for you; nothing is further from the truth! Have you noticed that everyone hits "rock bottom" at different levels of addiction? Some people get emphysema before they quit smoking, some are able to quit at a very early stage of addiction and some lose everything and die but never quit. That means that hitting "rock bottom" is not connected to disease and despair but to something else. What? What is that magic wand that returns people back to the fullness of life?

It is called THE POWER OF ADMITTING. In other words, facing the truth. This is the core of all the other 12

Step programs. Please try to understand clearly. The "rock bottom" happens when people honestly face that they lost control. Often a lifelong time of suffering happens before a person gets ready to admit. That shows that many people are scared of admitting the truth and don't understand why it is so important. Have you ever heard an alcoholic say, "Oh, I could stop drinking any time. I just don't want to." They don't want to admit they are out of control. That is called denial. Or have you heard a smoker say, "I could quit smoking but I really enjoy it and I feel fine." Do you see that this person is in denial? We all know that smoking is harmful to the body. Admitting creates a relief. By doing so we gain absolute clarity and there is no need to get into deep sorrow or become desperately ill in order to make a change. When we do admit that we have a problem, then we can start fixing this problem and that is when the shift happens. So let us hit rock bottom sooner than later. I will go first.

Hello, my name is Victoria Boutenko, and I am a cooked food addict and I have been clean for eight years. I relapsed only once, and though I don't want to eat cooked food right now, I know that if I would try cooked food then I would start eating and wanting cooked food. I know that about myself. I know that the desire for cooked food is a big giant sleeping somewhere in my body; sleeping right now, very soundly, it is not interfering with my experience of being completely alive and living my life fully. But I also know that I am a cooked food addict, and, that if I ate cooked food, this big giant could wake up and take over my life. There, I said it. I admitted to being a cooked food addict. The world is still here. No one fell over dead at my revelation. My husband still loves me. My children still love me. All is well. Admitting my addiction makes me stronger. I have labeled it. I know how to take care of myself because of identifying it. Power is in knowing oneself.

Cooked food is so addictive. If we go to the health store and we see an organic mango and it's -oh boy- $2.99 for one mango, we think, "How expensive!" Then we turn around to the deli and there are fresh baked croissants for $2.99. We think, "Oh boy, what a good deal, I'm hungry." We buy the croissant for an illusion of quick pleasure or to numb something empty inside. That's what we call unmanageability. How many of us have said, "I would really like to be a raw fooder, but when I come home and look in the fridge, I reach for the comfort food, not the raw food." Think about question two on the "Cooked Food Dependency Questionnaire." Do you eat late at night, even when you aren't hungry, just because your partner begins to unwrap something yummy? This is when we have lost control. You have decided not to eat late at night before bed, but you do it anyway because the temptation is there. The treat promises us some kind of pleasure. We remember times when the treat gave us pleasure, so we want it. This is addiction, when the want and need overrides your decision not to eat before bedtime. I've seen 132 people who had cancer, and they came to the health institute and they felt better. Their tumors shrank, and they decided to stay raw. They even applied to new jobs and applied to college. But when they went home, and Christmas came, they all failed. All of them died. They couldn't stay on raw food. They left children and loved ones behind because they couldn't resist the addiction to cooked food. That is the truth. I know their names. I knew those people. I was teaching them how to grow sprouts. I was talking to their families. Their families supported them. But they couldn't resist their addiction to cooked food and they died. I remember Cynthia from Michigan who had support from her whole family. She was a schoolteacher. Her three sons told her, "Mom, we're going to make juice for you. Just stay on this raw food diet and stay alive." Her husband said, "Stay raw, we all support you." She couldn't stay on the raw food diet. Her cancer came back. She died. Cooked food is addictive.

These stories from life show that the addiction to cooked food is stronger than the fear of death. It is stronger than the fear of disease, no matter how great the suffering and pain. The only way we can conquer cooked food is by understanding how addictive it is, by seeing that it has control over us and by using a 12 step program. Support is the most powerful force I know. If I didn't have support in my family, I would probably die. For a long time I didn't realize that in my home I had an AA group that gives me a hand whenever I feel weak. Yes, I've been 100% raw for eight years. I feel completely committed to eating raw. I have forgotten about cooked food. When I walk down the streets, I don't notice restaurants any more. When I go to Barnes and Noble I don't pay attention to the coffee smell. But I know that if I got hurt and I had go to the hospital where they don't have raw food, and I took a little bite, I know the outcome would be horrible. I've seen this happen to many of my friends. Something happened and they went back on cooked food, even though they had been strong, solid 100% raw fooders for a very long time. So I know for myself that addiction to cooked food is still in my body. The following fragment of sharing from a workshop demonstrates responses of different people to Step 1.

Linda: I think I hit rock bottom. I had been on raw foods for a very long time. During Christmas my family came around and I decided I wanted a traditional holiday. I wanted to do all the things I used to prepare. I did pumpkin pie and almond roca, and all these comfort foods that they loved and it gave me great pleasure in preparing for them. Anyway, I got very ill after the holidays from eating all that cooked food. That was my rock bottom.

Dalia: My eating is definitely unmanageable, and I definitely have an addiction to cooked foods, and I think it's because my parents introduced me to cooked foods at a very young age, and reinforced behavior with cooked food.

Carol: I'm having a hard time with this one.

Victoria: That is okay to have a hard time.

Carol: I guess I'm not at that point of admitting that I'm addicted.

Victoria: That's okay. Please feel welcome anyway.

Carol: I'm really wanting to move in that direction. But I'm struggling with talking about my addiction.

Victoria: I appreciate your sharing with us.

Bryan: I'm definitely addicted, and it's just unbelievable.

Kathleen: I've been on and off of raw foods for almost three years and I think it's really true that I am addicted. When I'm cooking tofu, or rice, or whatever for my family, I always know that I don't want to eat it, that I'd rather put energy into creating something raw. But I often end up eating cooked dishes with them.

CHAPTER NINE

Step Two

I believe that live vegan food is the most natural diet for a human being.

In Part One of this book, we have presented several reasons why raw food is the most natural diet for the human body. We discussed the importance of enzymes and how they relate to health. We discussed how the body has to adjust to cooked food by creating health-damaging mucus. We discussed the relationship between raw food and bacteria, parasites and disease.

In addition, I would like to share how raw food has changed the life of my family. Eight years ago we all became very sick. I had arrhythmia and was severely depressed. My husband suffered from painful arthritis. He had surgery scheduled for his hyperthyroid. My son was diagnosed with juvenile diabetes and was prescribed insulin. My daughter had asthma. All these illnesses are considered incurable by medical doctors. We also had many other problems like indigestion, obesity, lack of energy, mood swings, dental problems and others.

However, after we all went on a raw diet, all four of us got completely cured. Today we experience radiant health and constant happiness. I believe that our health is beyond what most people experience. We don't have any medical insurance because we feel totally in charge of our health. We continually experience a high level of energy. Each one of us can run for many miles. In 1998 we hiked across the United States on the Pacific Crest Trail. Other people may have doubts, but we know all the changes in our health started to happen when we went on raw food.

CHAPTER TEN

Step Three

**I shall gain necessary skills,
learn basic raw recipes and obtain
equipment to prepare live food.**

How important is tasty raw food? We have agreed earlier that for most people eating is a first pleasure in life. Therefore most people WILL NOT stay on a raw diet if the food is not delicious. Can the raw food be as tasty as cooked food? Absolutely! I have learned how to prepare very delicious raw food, and my family has been successfully teaching secrets of raw gourmet dishes to hundreds of men and women of different ages. During the last few years I simply stopped telling people that my food is raw unless they asked.

Once a woman called me and asked, "I heard you are a good cook. Can you cater for a wedding, for 50 people?" She did not ask for a raw wedding, but at that particular time I was not in a position to refuse the extra cash. So I said, "Sure." I had so much fun preparing a 3-tier wedding cake, appetizers, soups, salads, portabella mushroom burgers, sundaes and ice creams! There were no raw fooders at that wedding. All

guests were accustomed to a Standard American Diet (SAD).
Nobody complained! The only question everybody asked
was, "How come everything is so delicious?" Guests loved the
food and they wanted to meet the chef. When I announced to
everybody that all the food was raw and vegan, all people
were very surprised "that healthy food could be so tasty."

You're not going to turn into a raw chef just by watching, as you cannot turn into a good swimmer by watching
Olympic swimmers. In order to learn how to swim, you
need to get wet, and cold, and get some water in your nose.
If you want to become a good raw gourmet chef, you need
to unpack your new blender, processor, juicer and dehydrator and place them on the counter in your kitchen. Don't
just own them, use them, jump in and get messy. Get your
hands sticky. Spill the contents from the Vita-Mix all over
the kitchen. It's unavoidable, so the sooner the better.
Experiment, have fun. If your creation doesn't taste good
yet, put it in your compost. All earthworms from your
neighborhood will gather into your garden attracted by
your cuisine. You can only learn by trial and error how to
make delicious food.

For five years my daughter Valya was afraid to make frosting for the cake. She said, "I won't make it. It won't taste
good." Once I was out of town and our close friend asked
Valya to prepare a cake for a birthday. My daughter had to
make the entire cake by herself and she did. When I got
home Valya told me "It was so easy! You just take nuts, dates
and water, and blend it, and it's a frosting! If you want you
can create different flavors by adding vanilla, or carob, or
lemon peel or other natural ingredients, but it's so simple!"
Valya showed me a good dozen cute little teacakes with

different frostings on them. She was talking about this for the entire day. "It's so simple!" she said.

My husband Igor was afraid to make live gardenburgers. He said, "It was easy with real meat, you just cut a piece and fry it with oil. But now I am supposed to create a meat from carrots without a cow?" He saw me preparing live gardenburger hundreds of times but he was afraid that it was too complicated for him. For six years he never even tried to make one. Then we had an emergency situation when too many people showed up for a dinner. I was busy preparing soup. Who will make gardenburgers? Igor didn't have a choice. So he did it! Even before I finished making soup he was done. Since then I have never made another live gardenburger. Igor took over. Now we call this dish "Igorburger."

Igor started to enjoy preparing raw food more and more. He created many of his own dishes. His Russian Borodinsky crackers are popular all over the world. In Iceland Igor was demonstrating how to create a raw sandwich. He put live gardenburgers on crackers and decorated with dry olives and paprika. When people tried his raw sandwiches they were amazed how delicious Igor's sandwiches were. One woman exclaimed, "This sandwich is worth living for!"

If you want to learn how to prepare delicious raw meals, please read attentively the rest of this chapter. There is a principal difference between cooking meals and preparing live food. The following table will help you to understand why in preparing raw dishes we cannot rely on recipes.

Comparison of cooking and preparing

- Ingredients in cooked food always change their initial taste as a result of cooking.

- Ingredients in raw food never change their initial taste.

- Cooked food has pale unattractive colors and textures.

- Raw food is very colorful and naturally appealing to human eyes.

- The original rich flavors of raw fruits, vegetables, nuts and seeds disappear almost completely after being heated.

- The original rich flavors of raw fruits, vegetables, nuts and seeds stay in the food after preparing without heating.

- Plain cooked food is tasteless, requiring enhancement with salt, pepper and other condiments.

- Raw food is naturally delicious and requires very little or no condiments.

- The taste of cooked food is determined by condiments.

- The taste of raw food is determined by a bouquet of tastes of main ingredients.

- Condiments have permanent taste.

- Raw fruits, vegetables, nuts and seeds have wide spectrums of tastes.

- When making cooked food, to follow a recipe is the most important.

- When preparing a raw dish, following a recipe doesn't guarantee a delicious result. You need to always adjust the final taste.

follow every step, measure everything and turn out with something different each time because of the variables inherent in live food. Cooked corn, cooked zucchini, cooked peas and other cooked vegetables taste almost the same and require oil and salt added, at the least. Raw corn, zucchini, peas and other raw vegetables, all have their own unique taste that is impossible to confuse. When I prepare a raw dish I use recipes only as ideas, as general guidelines or just for the ingredients. Then I adjust the final taste using a method of five tastes. There are thousands of different tastes in natural food but if we could balance five major ones, the food will be so delicious that everyone will say, "Wow!" These five tastes are: sweet, sour, salty, spicy and bitter. When you learn to balance the five tastes, you will make delicious food. When all five groups of the taste buds on your tongue are excited you will say, "Wow!"

When you attempt to un-cook a delicious meal, make sure that all five tastes are present in the final taste and not even one is missing. People who have been preparing raw gourmet meals everyday for many months, definitely could tell if one or two ingredients are missing by just tasting food once or twice. Others have to taste freshly made meals five times, asking each time a very simple question: Is it spicy enough? Is it salty enough? Is it sweet enough? Is it sour enough? Is it bitter enough? The five tastes don't have to be strong but just enough for a particular dish. For example, the strongest tastes in a gardenburger should be sweet, spicy and salty with only a touch of sour and bitter, but all five have to be present. Otherwise the gardenburger will taste bland.

Usually, when you have just prepared a dish and go through your first round of five-spoon tasting, two or three tastes are missing. Add ingredients for the missing tastes, mix again and start five spoon tasting all over again. Continue until the five major tastes are balanced in the nice bouquet. I call this process "adjusting the taste." In the beginning adjusting can take longer than preparing. Don't be discouraged, your pace will speed up with practice. At the same time your raw food will become unbeatable.

Whether you prepare a cake, a dressing or a nut cutlet, the bouquet of all five tastes needs to be present. We, for some reason, have this idea that if food is already healthy, it doesn't have to be delicious. So we throw the celery and lemon juice into the blender and mix and we don't even taste it. But when we begin to eat, it may be unbearably bitter or too sour. That's why we use the taste test and add what is missing.

After approximately one and a half years of consuming 100% raw food you will start noticing that you prefer to eat whole food rather than prepared, more and more often. As a matter of fact, all whole foods, if they are ripe, already have the most balanced bouquet of taste in them naturally. However, their taste is so delicate that unfortunately, after many years of consuming cooked food filled with condiments, our taste buds cannot enjoy natural taste. That is why we need a transition time.

The following is a list of suggested ingredients for five taste groups. This is only a fraction of what is available on planet Earth. Many plants possess different tastes but have one or two that are dominate. You have to apply common sense and not add vanilla to the soup or garlic to the candy. Please be creative, these are just ideas for you.

For a sour taste add: Lemons, rhubarb, lemon grass, sour grass, sorrel, tomatoes, rejuvelac, nut or seed yogurt or apple cider vinegar.

For a sweet taste add: Dry fruit such as figs, dates, prunes, raisins; fresh fruits such as ripe banana, mango, peach, pear; apple juice, orange juice, raw honey or fresh stevia leaves.

For a spicy taste add: Garlic leaves or cloves, onion leaves or bulbs, ginger, mustard greens or seeds, radish, horseradish, cayenne pepper, wasabe sea weed, herbs fresh or dry such as basil, dill, cilantro, rosemary, cinnamon, nutmeg, vanilla or peppermint.

For a salty taste add: Celery, cilantro, dill, parsley, sea vegetables such as dulce, kelp, nori, arame or Celtic sea salt.

For a bitter taste add: Parsley, celery tops, endive, garlic, onion, dandelion, bay leaf, sage, poultry seasoning or cayenne pepper.

CHAPTER ELEVEN

Step Four

I shall live in harmony with people who eat cooked food.

I have a question for you. What emotions do you feel when someone is telling you what to do? You probably had many instances in your life when another person was giving you advice and you didn't agree. What was your reaction? Can you remember a time when a friend said to you something like, "Gary, you need to start jogging. You're getting fat." Or, "Tom, you should cut off these dread locks." Or, "Paula, you should stop smoking. You have children." Did these suggestions help you? Probably not. Remember when you were a kid and your mom or your dad said, "You're running around in the streets too much, you really need to read more books." How did you feel? Did you feel drawn to books immediately? Did you say, "Oh, thank you, Dad, I'll go and read right now?" Chances are you felt rebellious and resentful and the last thing you wanted to do was to go pick up a book, sit down and read. Here are what my students said in the class about their response to other people's "unsolicited helpful suggestions."

Nancy: I would breathe a little smile, but of course I wouldn't do it.

George: I just smile and ignore.

Dorothy: I would feel resistance, and I hate that feeling. I would hate being forced and I'd have to start being dishonest.

Bryan: I'd feel really sarcastic.

Whitney: I wouldn't do it, because it's not their choice. I'd have resistance.

Wendy: I want to please. I want to do what they ask me to do, but then I'll be secretive about it, and be resentful.

Carla: Depression, so bad.

Sam: Sometimes when they think I should change something even if I know it's right, I won't do it, but I'll get mad that I know it's right and I'm not doing it. I get a little bit of anger too.

When someone tells us that they know better than we do what is good for us, we tend to feel angry and upset, like they're trying to control us. We feel annoyed, negative, and we shut them and their advice out. We feel attacked, hurt and uncomfortable.

That is precisely how your family is going to feel if you come home and show off and say, "I am raw now." An announcement of a family member to be a raw fooder can be a frightening thing for the rest of the family. Cooked food is what we all know and consider normal and expected in our culture. Do you want those you love to feel rebellious, negative, shut off, controlled or angry? This is exactly how they will feel if you tell them one day, "I'm going to be raw now, so don't eat that crap in front of me! Just the look of it makes me sick!"

We need to do just the opposite. When you decide to become raw, talk to your family as soon as possible. Explain to them, "You know darling, this is not about you. Eating raw food is the choice I am making for myself. I'm not asking you to eat raw food. It's really okay with me that you continue to drink beer and smoke your cigarettes, and eat your favorite steak. I love you the way you are. It's me who's trying to change. It's not about you. I don't expect you to follow me, to be interested, or even to try my food." Don't wait until your family asks if it's okay to eat cooked food in front of you. Go ahead and talk to them right away. Watch how they will sigh with relief.

We don't even have to speak to make those we love uncomfortable. Some of us throw certain glances that convey the same meaning as the words discussed previously. For example, a woman in one of my classes said to me, "My family is angry with my raw foodism even though I never pushed anybody to eat raw food. My husband has been vegan for 30 years. My son is 12 and they always ask me to prepare cooked meals. When I cook food for them I go off my raw food diet. I don't feel much support. My son makes all kinds of jokes about my green juices, and he wonders why I have to eat my cake with a spoon." I said to her, "You might be doing something that irritates them that you're not aware of. Just watch yourself, and catch those moments. Don't watch others. Watch and see what you are doing to antagonize your family." The next week she came to class and said, "Yeah. I caught myself several times poking little pins in certain painful places. I'd say something hurtful or look disgusted or put out. I changed my attitude toward my family, and they, in turn, shifted toward me and it only took one week. When I started accepting them, then they accepted me back. Now my husband is making juice every morning and bringing it to me in bed. He says, 'Honey, I want you to stay on raw food.' Suddenly my house has become a peaceful place, and my son is willing to try everything I make."

I am making my living by teaching raw food classes and I have been on a 100% raw food diet for eight years. But if somebody had told me ten years ago to go raw, I would have been so mad. I wasn't ready. Cooked food is addictive. Giving up cooked food isn't easy. Everyone must choose their own time.

Another example is my friend Tina from Denver. She had a serious health problem. For many months she had to go to the hospital to undergo a procedure that was very embarrassing and painful for her. When we came to town to visit, she saw what we were eating and she was interested. She asked, "Can you show me how to do it? I'm willing to try because I have surgery (a colostomy) scheduled in two weeks which I would rather not do." Within a matter of days, she started to have normal bowel movements. She went on raw food for good. She avoided the surgery. Tina understood that for her, there were only two choices: raw food, no surgery, life and health, or cooked food, colostomy and eventually death. Tina chose life. At the time of our visit, Tina's four children were major junk food eaters and her husband enjoyed vodka, steak, pork chops and pig's fat, which he used like bologna. Tina did not tell her family that she was going raw. She kept cooking for them as she always did. She said, "I'm going to keep it quiet." I agreed with her. I said, "Don't even mention it to them. Don't irritate them. Let them just leave you alone. Tell them that you don't expect them to do anything." Tina didn't mention her diet change to them. One year passed. We were driving through Denver and we stopped by. I saw Tina's husband, Sam, and he looked different. I said, "Sam, is something wrong? You have changed." He replied with a grin, "I became 100% raw one month ago. The family is all happy and the children are raw, too." I asked, "What happened?" Sam told me the story of why he became raw. He said that one day, about a month ago, he'd gone to pick up Tina at work. He arrived a little early and sat down within view of her desk to wait. He noticed that his wife was so beautiful. He saw the customers flirting with his wife. He was looking at her through new eyes. He saw how she'd gotten so healthy, sexy and beautiful. All of a sudden he felt so inadequate. He said, "I ran to the restroom and I looked at myself. I saw puffs under my eyes and a red face and gray hairs sticking up all over. I opened my shirt, and I looked at these pimples all over my chest. Nobody is going to flirt with me." He told me that he realized Tina had been getting healthy and beautiful and he had just been aging. Sam decided he needed to make a change so he could keep up with his wife. He said, "On the way back home I begged her to please help me to become raw like you." Tina was happy to help her husband become raw. Tina told me that as soon as Sam went raw, the children said they wanted to be raw too! Her daughter became thin and beautiful and was now taking part in an audition for the theater. Everything was just going wonderfully. Tina said that she felt a call from God, and things happened like never before in their life. Tina is a very wise woman. She didn't say a word to her family about becoming raw. She made her food and enjoyed it without putting any expectations on her family. Her body healed and her family observed the changes.

Because of her good example, her family made the choice to follow.

I can give you many similar examples that show the importance of living in peace with people who eat cooked food. Do you understand how important it is? It is crucial! What do we do in our real life? We do the opposite. We ruin the peace around ourselves. We start the war. We make people irritated with raw food. Please make a conscious choice to live in peace with all around you. You can do this. This in when the miracles happen. When people are not afraid that you are going to put any pressure on them, they are willing to cooperate. We have no right to control others. We have no right to expect other people to change when they are not ready. We have no right to tell them what to do. In fact, our duty is to explain to others that we don't expect them to change.

Does that mean that there won't be any more family dinners? Why not? Go home, sit down with your partner, and say, "Honey, let's have a family dinner. You enjoy your pork chops and I'll enjoy my stuffed bell pepper. We'll talk about our day and we'll enjoy our time together." After all, family is about love. Family is not about food. When your loved ones know that you are not expecting anything from them, they can relax around you. They can support you without feeling pressured to change. We raw fooders have made a choice for ourselves for serious reasons. We made the right choice for us, not the right choice for everyone.

When I went on raw food I did just the opposite of my advice to you. I went around telling everyone to go on raw food. I was chasing overweight ladies in Safeway, trying to explain to them how easy it is to lose weight. I was so excited about the healthy changes my family was experiencing, I got carried away. I made a lot of enemies before I understood that people need to find their own way and decide their own path.

When we respect other people's rights we can ask for support from our loved ones. We need to be sincere and not be afraid to tell them, "My darling, please help me. I need support. I need to eat raw food for my health, because when I eat cooked food I feel as if I'm falling apart. When I eat raw food, I feel more energy and I have more love for you. Please help me. I don't need you to be raw. I have an idea. Instead of buying me chocolates on Sunday, will you buy me a ripe mango? Or any exotic fruit would be a great pleasure for me. I so appreciate your thoughtfulness. Those cookies that we have in the house, it would be so helpful to me if you'd keep them in your truck so that I can't eat them in a moment of weakness. I appreciate your support so much."

Be firm with your friends, co-workers and all your relatives. If you are not firm they will continue to offer you cooked food. Be vulnerable and tell your family and close friends, "Listen I need your help. It's very important for me and my health now, that I go on raw food. Without your help I cannot do it. Support me, don't offer me any cooked food. You can eat absolutely whatever you want but don't offer it to me please." To ask for support is different than to ask them to go on raw food. People would love to be supportive, because we usually have love in our families and among friends.

Millie is a good example. When Millie was diagnosed with breast cancer, she started raw food. Her whole family, three big sons and her husband, were hostile and just hated the word "raw." Then Millie attended the 12 Step class. With Step Four in mind, she went through and rearranged her communication with her family. I heard from her via email some weeks after the class. She said, "My husband is growing proud of me! Everything worked just miraculously! My family now understands that I need support." Because she has cancer, they understand she needs support, and since she doesn't want or demand them to be raw, she doesn't put pressure on them. They feel very balanced and in peace.

No matter how we would love the rest of the family to benefit from raw food, we can control only one person in the world, ourselves. It is not our business to control our children or our parents, even if they are dying from cancer. I learned my lesson when my mother was dying from cancer and I flew all the way to Russia to put her on raw food so she would survive. I was working very hard, going to the farmers market, buying carrots and juicing them all day long. On the third day as soon as I left to the market, my mother whispered to my brother, "Can you make me some scrambled eggs? I'm starving!" When I returned my mother's room was filled with the smell of scrambled eggs. My brother said, "I don't want to lie to you. She asked for it." At that minute I felt how cruel it was for me to push my mother. If she really is not ready, what good does it do? We have already discussed how we feel when someone tells us something we are not ready for.

I know one young man from Seattle who told me that he is really sorry for his mother who is suffering from tremendous pain. He told me that he and his mother are the closest people in the world. He said, "I wish she would go on raw food so she wouldn't have to suffer." I asked him, "Do you know how you make her suffer even more from feeling that she is not meeting your expectation?" He said, "I never thought of that." After he gave it a thought, he came home, and told his mother, "You know, it's okay with me if you're not going to try my diet." In a few days he called me back and said, "A miracle happened, Mom wanted to try my food!"

I met people who started to push their family on raw food even before they tried raw diet themselves. Like Linda and Jim. After Linda visited just one raw food class she came home and demanded Jim go on raw food. She came to the next class and complained that her husband didn't support her. Somehow she dragged Jim to the last class. He had already developed strong prejudice and resistance towards raw food. After listening to the lecture, Jim became very interested. In two months Jim called me and told that he has been 100% raw for two months but Linda found it challenging and went back to eating cooked food.

If people around you have any suspicion that you will try to make them raw, they will criticize you to make you go off raw food. Don't argue with them and don't try to prove scientifically that you are right. Instead you may tell them, "I am deeply moved by your concern about me but believe me, I feel very well. As always, food will continue to unite us. Now you will eat your plate and I will eat mine, and we will still eat together." When you make your food, don't just put a bunch of sprouts on your plate because your partner will think you are deprived of pleasures. Make yourself some very nice looking dish. Later, your friends and partners will be drawn to try some of your food because it looks so nice. Then they will try it once and say, "It's not bad."

Sometimes raw fooders put extremely high pressure on their loved ones demanding them to change. In Phoenix Arizona, three anti-raw husbands united and organized a club for oppressed husbands of raw food wives. They meet once a week and eat a cooked pizza. Hopefully this chapter will prevent the need for more organizations such as this.

What about the children in your house that you need to prepare meals for? We have already hooked our children on cooked foods, and we have to slowly increase the ratio of raw food to cooked food. Have plenty of raw fruits and vegetables handy for snacks. Learn how to make live ice creams, nut milks, nut-milk shakes, smoothies, live candies, cakes and other kid-friendly foods. Show them raw food can be wonderful. Invite your children into preparing raw food together. Buy them a cheap blender at a garage sale. But the most important, be a good example and don't make a big fuss about raw foods. Remember, kids learn what they see. Show them harmony and love around the table. We can all sit together and enjoy one another's company. Family is not about food.

I am often asked how to not insult the relatives who associate food with love and to refuse their food is disrespectful to them. To answer that, I will say that next time we meet I will bring a huge gallon of vodka, and if you don't drink it with me right away, while standing up with a toast for health, you disrespect me, as a native Russian. I assume that most of you will have no problem find my correct words for refusing my offer without insulting me.

When I went to Russia and refused traditional Russian food my relatives felt offended for a while, but then when they knew how serious raw food was to me and my health, they weren't offended any more. Yes, I did lose some people's friendships, but gained so many more other friendships. My family in Russia didn't completely understand what I was doing. They thought I was turning into a crazy capitalist or something. But when they knew how important raw food was to me, because they love me and I love them, I was able to explain to them that it's for my health. I showed them my picture before and after. When I looked quite different two years apart, they could tell I really was better off than I was before. They never knew that I could look so good. How to avoid insulting the relatives? It's up to you. You will be able to find this out if you are really looking for answers.

If there is a loving atmosphere in the family, we can always work things out. Eight years ago when I first told my husband that I wanted to try to go on raw food for two months, he told me, "No way, I'm a Russian man, I'm used to Russian borscht with its fragrance of beef and pork and spices." He said, "Food unites people and if you're going to go on this diet alone, you'll see, we're going to get divorced." That was his first reaction. I understood where my husband came from. But I knew that if the raw food was really important for me, I would find the words to explain how I felt that there was no life for me without raw food. I clearly felt that raw food was a solution for me because I was literally dying. Raw food gave me a big hope of survival. I knew that I would find words to explain this.

CHAPTER TWELVE

Step Five

I shall stay away from temptations.

Imagine a raw island where all people are raw fooders. There are no smells of cooked food on the street, no stoves or ovens in the kitchens, nobody cooks their food and all the restaurants serve only live cuisine. The billboards ask, "Got wheat-grass juice?" and all children get baskets of exotic fruits for Halloween. Wouldn't it be easy for us to live on raw food there? Why is that easy on the raw island and hard in our real life? There are no temptations on the raw island and our real life is penetrated with them.

Let us first gain clarity on the word "temptation." What is temptation? Please try to find answers by yourself. I will help you with a series of questions. Is there a difference between temptation and desire? Temptation includes desire but what else is there? When we desire to eat a cucumber or if we want to pet a puppy, we don't expect anything bad to happen, right? As far as we know. We don't call it temptation, we call it desire. When do we call desire "temptation?" What does the word "temptation" have, that the word "desire" doesn't? Please try to think so that you have complete clarity about temptation. Let's go to the root. We have to discover. Is there anything negative in temptation at all? We know we shouldn't have it. Why? We call temptation something that we know is going to hurt us. In the long run, we will have either pain or disease or death or other problems. Sounds awful, but why is that tempting? Because it promises us pleasure in the short term. How quickly do we experience pleasure? Instantly. How quickly does the punishment happen? In the long run, sometimes it feels like never.

So, temptation is a desire for something that promises us pleasure in the short term with the awareness of negative consequences later. We anticipate fast pleasure. This pleasure is so dear to us that we get tempted. Now that we clearly understand what temptation is and how it is different from desire, we can learn how to successfully avoid temptation.

Do you believe that you can fight temptation by your will power? I, personally, don't know anybody who can stand temptations. I only meet people who know how to avoid temptations. That is why it's best for us not to be exposed to temptations.

There are two kinds of temptations, avoidable and unavoidable. I consider avoidable temptations those that you can realistically stay away from for at least a couple of months. I call temptations unavoidable if you cannot control their presence.

Do you know what your biggest temptations are in a field of cooked food? They are always based on your personal weaknesses to some cooked dishes. Many students in my classes named one or more of the following: Coffee, chocolate, corn chips, baked potato, popcorn, candies, cheese, bread, pizza, pasta, rice, cookies, cake, and potato chips.

Most people are aware of their weaknesses. If you have trouble figuring out which cooked food could possibly tempt you, the following questions might help. Which part of the cooked life will you miss most of all? Which cooked food could possibly make you slip off the raw diet? What is the most frightening for you in going on raw food? Knowing our biggest temptations helps us to become aware of the places of temptations. I'd like to give you two examples.

Say your biggest temptation is popcorn. Then the places of temptations for you are the movie theaters and sometimes other public places. I classify this temptation as avoidable. Of course, if you have a popcorn machine at your work place, then I would call it unavoidable.

If your biggest temptation is coffee, then the places of temptations are: Coffee shops, such as Starbucks, all deli shops, all gas stations, some parties, some offices, even Barnes & Noble Book Stores and many other public places. I consider this temptation unavoidable.

Do this exercise. Honestly try to remember all your temptations in the field of cooked food. Write them down. If there are too many of them, group them in categories. Then take two pieces of paper. On one sheet write "avoidable temptations" on the other "unavoidable temptations." Draw a vertical line on both pages. List your temptations on the left side. On the right side of each temptation write down all the places of temptation you can think of. This exercise makes you aware of all the places where you could be tempted, so you could get prepared to meet the challenge.

Let us first discuss avoidable temptations. Some examples of avoidable temptations are pasta, cake, chocolate, specific

national food, all kinds of chips, unless, of course, you work
at the factory that manufactures this food. When you decide
to go on raw food, make a serious and conscious effort not to
be exposed to these cooked products for about two months
or longer in order to build up a resistance. Learn to substitute
those foods with raw food dishes. Take all tempting cooked
foods out of your house, office and car. Don't leave a hidden
stash of your favorite cooked food in the house, because the
thought of it will be chasing you until you eat it, you won't
be able to relax or concentrate on work. When we are hungry, angry, lonely or depressed, we think that eating our
favorite food will help to numb us out and give us pleasure.

Avoid advertisements as much as you can for about two
months. Have you ever noticed that when advertisers pro-
mote drinking, they portray a good time where everyone is
smiling. The advertisers leave out the negative consequences
of drinking such as hangovers, throwing up and fights.
Magazines and TV are filled with advertisements of cooked
or processed food. Most of the ads connect cooked food to
happy social events. The idea is that if you eat the product
advertised, you'll be as happy and fulfilled as the people
appear to be in the ad. We all know the ad is staged and the
people are just actors, but we still crave the food and the
FEELING in the ad.

Don't go to parties until you become firm. Go to raw
food classes and potlucks instead. Spend your free time prac-
ticing how to prepare new raw food dishes. Later, when you
will learn how to put together a couple of raw gourmet dishes, you could become a party celebrity as have many other
raw fooders.

Feed yourself well before you go shopping so you won't

be tempted by all the food screaming at you. Try to avoid
stores that hand out free samples of food at every aisle. If you
have to go there, stuff your mouth with raisins, nuts or raw
crackers. Keep your mouth busy with raw food and shake
your head "NO" when offered samples. The toughest time
usually lasts about two months. Do what you can to survive
on raw food through that time. Read some books on drugs. I
found that helpful. Create a raw island around yourself.
Remember, what is impossible in the presence of temptations
becomes very easy and enjoyable in a temptation-free zone.

Now let us talk about unavoidable temptations. Some
examples of unavoidable temptations are: Cooked food that
other members of your family eat, vending machines at your
office, a bakery across the street that smells every morning,
free coffee at your work, delicious presents from your friends,
free food samples at the store or in the mail, pizza day at
school, business lunches, free candies at your bank, bulk food
bins in the store, free cookies at your church, family reunions
and many others.

When we were dealing with avoidable temptations, our
main strategy was to withdraw ourselves from being exposed
to them. There is no way to apply the same strategy to the
unavoidable temptations. What else can we do? Use our dis-
cipline and will power? We have already mentioned that we
cannot overcome temptations with will power. When we
don't see temptations we are sure that we can stand them just
fine by our will power. But in reality, when we are actually
facing temptation, we fail again.

However, we can prepare ourselves psychologically to
handle unavoidable temptations without indulging in them.
In order to know what to say in a situation when somebody

unexpectedly is offering us a tempting food, we have to think
ahead of time what we are going to say, how we are going to
react to that.

I teach a game in my classes that helps people to deal with
unavoidable temptations. By playing this game students practice saying "No" to temptations with grace. First students identify their weakness. Then we role-play different situations
where they might be offered these foods. When unexpectedly
offered their favorite cooked food, people have to know ahead
of time what they will say. The following is an example of
playing this game during one of the workshops. Lara volun-
teered to play the role of the "tempted" because she wants to
stop drinking coffee. Now Lara is standing in front of the class.

Victoria: Lara, are you sure that you want to quit drinking coffee?

Lara: Oh yes, I have been promising myself to quit for
two years and the longest I was able to go without it was a
week. Just enough for the headache to pass.

Victoria: Lara, what is your favorite brand of coffee and
where do you usually get it?

Lara: Latté. I buy it myself at Starbucks.

Victoria to students: Please make tempting offers to Lara.
Be creative, so that your offer sounds real and hard to refuse.

Victoria to Lara: Lara, you will have to say, "No, thank
you," plus you have to do it in such a way that you don't put
people down. In a real situation, when somebody is whole-
heartedly giving you something, you don't tell them, "Get out
of here, I don't drink coffee." Sincerely express your appreciation for their thoughtfulness and make an alternative offer
like, "Thank you very much, I am really touched, but can we
drink juice instead?" If they insist, stay firm, tell them, "Sorry,

I cannot drink coffee any more, I have health problems." Or say, "I have decided to quit drinking coffee." Or, "My doctor doesn't let me."

Karen: Lara, guess what! I was at the Starbucks, they have an amazing sale there, and I bought you your favorite coffee Latte. Here!

Lara: Oh my God . . .

Victoria to Lara: What do you say?

Lara: Oh, Karen, this is so nice of you! Thank you! But I don't drink coffee anymore. I have high blood pressure. But thank you! Do you think you could find somebody else who might enjoy it?

Karen: Sure! I understand.

Mike: I am your father. Congratulations! You have inherited a black coffee factory from us, your parents. You are wealthy now. According to our old tradition, every morning you will taste the company's fresh coffee.

Lara: Mmm, thank you father, I am so moved! But my doctor is seriously concerned about my blood pressure. Do you think we could let our manager try the coffee? Or maybe I could symbolically hold the cup without drinking it?

Mike: I understand, daughter. We'll work something out.

Sarah: Hey, Lara, I am so glad that I have you as a friend, because I have just won a certificate from Starbucks! For a year one can get free coffee of any kind. And you know that I don't drink coffee. So I am giving it to you! Ta-ta!

Lara: That sounds so great! Thank you so much! But you know, Sarah, you are my good friend and you will understand me. I have decided not to drink coffee any more for health reasons. But I bet you can think of someone else to give such a gift.

Sarah: Okay.

Jerry: Lara, we have been driving with you for several hours, it's 2:00 a.m. and we both feel sleepy, but we have to drive. Let us stop at the gas station and I will buy for us some coffee so we could continue driving.

Lara: Thank you, Jerry, I don't mind if you buy coffee for yourself, but I know from my experience that coffee wouldn't help me anyway. So I would rather take a little nap while you are buying coffee. Maybe I could munch on some almonds.

Marlene: Hi, Lara, are you ready for our monthly meeting at a coffee shop? I have so much news to tell you! Let's go.

Lara: I am sorry, Marlene, but I cannot go to the coffee shop.

Marlene: How can you say that? Are you not my friend any more?

Lara: Oh, Marlene, of course I am your friend and I cannot wait to hear everything, but my doctor doesn't let me drink coffee anymore. If I will go to the coffee shop I might be tempted. Let us go to a juice bar instead and I will treat you to a nice smoothie.

Marlene: But we have always met there, it won't be the same!

Lara: Listen, Marlene, I don't mean to offend you. You are my best friend and I need your support now. Please understand me.

Marlene: Okay, let's go for a smoothie.

Victoria: Lara, can you please share with the group about any shifting inside of you during our game? Do you feel more empowered now?

Lara: I am truly amazed how real I felt. It was hard for me to say no, especially in the beginning. Then it became easier and easier. I can tell now that this was my first time when I really was going to say no. Before this moment I have never even realistically thought about this. I feel like I have paved my way. Now I have a whole repertoire to draw from in real situations. Thank you all for your creative effort.

All my students find this game very helpful because it gives ideas for many tough situations. I recommend to play it in support groups and at the raw potlucks. Everyone should have a chance to play at least once.

Scientists who do research about drugs and addictive substances talk about a chain reaction. The reaction is harder to stop if we haven't decided beforehand how we will choose to act. For example, when an alcoholic has money in his pocket to pay the rent, but he meets his friend on the corner, he is much more likely to follow that friend into a bar and spend the rent money on drinks. That's called the chain reaction. When you see the vending machine, you're going to go into a chain reaction of wanting what you see unless you have already figured out your response. The safest time to figure out how you will react is when you are at home or at a place where there are no possible temptations. This is the time to figure out what you are going to do.

Now go back to your paper of unavoidable temptations that you face in your life. On the right side across from each temptation, write down your ideas or strategies on how to deal with them. For example, you could decide to stuff your mouth with raisins before you get near the vending machine. Or if you live in a home where you are the only one on raw food, you might designate a part of your kitchen as a temptation-free zone.

When you have built some resistance, I want to encourage

you to go out to the restaurants. You don't have to sit home feeling isolated forever. To socialize is important. In the beginning to go out with a friend would be easier. If you have three or four raw food friends you may go out together once a week. Decide where you will meet, and then call ahead to reserve a table. Everybody brings their own dressing, and you all have a super time socializing and eating delicious raw food. In addition, somebody can bring raw crackers or little sprouted seeds to put on top of everyone's salad and you all sit down and enjoy your time together in the restaurant. We all need social pleasure.

If you don't yet know how to make delicious dressing, mix equal proportions of Bragg's Liquid Aminos with good oil and apple cider vinegar, shake it well and that's your dressing. Have it always in the car. This dressing will stay fresh for a long time. Take it to the restaurant, pour on top of your salad and enjoy your meal.

To make going out easier and more enjoyable I recommend that you use the wonderful card that my friend Jonathan put together. Copy the following card on a hard paper, cut it and keep in your wallet. When I go out to the restaurant alone or with friends, I don't have to feel embarrassed in front of everybody trying to explain to the frightened waitress my special request. Instead I handle her a card with a smile. I think all the chefs appreciate a chance to be creative because my dishes always come so beautiful.

Jonathan's Card

I EAT ONLY RAW, UNCOOKED FOODS.
I would like a salad or vegetable plate
with only fresh, uncooked items:

lettuce	tomato	avocado	carrot
zucchini	sprouts	cucumber	celery
broccoli	scallions	radish	onion
cauliflower	parsley	cabbage	kale
spinach	cilantro	bell pepper	beets
mushrooms	bok choy	arugula	chard

Thank you for your creative efforts!

Unfortunately, there are very few places that serve organic food. Still I think that to go out once a week with your friends is better than to be so lonely that you will go and eat pizza. You won't get off your diet by eating an inorganic salad once a week. In fact, having the social interaction will support you in maintaining a raw food lifestyle.

By going out you will get used to being exposed to temptations and not thinking about them. You cannot always be cocooned in your own house. Sometime you have to step outside and be able to handle that.

After a couple of months of staying away from temptations, you will notice that you stopped paying attention to the restaurants and any raw food in general. You might also get an illusion that your addiction to cooked food is over and you can eat or try small pieces of cooked food once in a while. When you will try a bite of cooked food once, you might not feel much. But on the next morning you might notice that you will begin to think about cooked food and to pay attention to whatever cooked food you'll see. If you will give into temptation once more, you might lose peace of mind. Then you would have to start all over. We described a story of our relapse in our book *Raw Family*.

CHAPTER THIRTEEN

Step Six

I shall create support for myself.

In simple words, find yourself a "raw buddy." All you need to do is to find one person in your block, in your household or at your work with whom you meet daily to talk and share a meal together. This step might seem to you as not important and hard to fulfill. From my point of view, personal support is crucial both for the beginning of your raw foodism and for the long term. Becoming a raw fooder without personal support seems to me next to impossible. At the same time, staying raw with support is fun and easy.

The most important is that your buddy is supportive of what you are doing. You may call this person your support group, your buddy, raw brother, raw sister anything you like. If you are really dedicated, I know you will find the right person for support. Everybody in my 12 Steps classes found a support person. In some cases, the buddy is not even a raw fooder. It could be a relative who is supportive of the dear one who has an illness. For example, Aneta has cancer, and her husband, who is not a raw fooder, decided to be her buddy.

How does support work? Almost always, psychologically, other people's opinions are more important for us than our own. To break the commitment we made to other people is much harder for us than to break the commitment we made to ourselves.

For example, when you go to a salad bar at a restaurant, you could talk yourself into eating something cooked. Your mind says, "Who knows for sure if the beans are really cooked, so go ahead and put them on your plate. And these beets, they could be raw. They may be just fermented. Fermentation is good for you. So put it on your plate also. And this mayonnaise is less than one percent of your meal, so it's OK." But when you go to the salad bar with your friend who is aware and supportive of your effort, then your mind shuts up and behaves. The most ideal situation is to share at least one meal a day with this person. Please don't think that it is too hard to do. You are having at least three meals a day anyway. Why not share breakfast, lunch, dinner or a snack with your buddy?

When dining alone, you can say, "Oh, I am too tired to prepare a meal, I will just eat an apple." When there are two of you gathering for a dinner you will have to prepare something more attractive. Sometimes you might become more inspired and create a special meal. Nicer dining will make your raw life more pleasant.

One person is limited in time and energy, and cannot dehydrate, grow sprouts, make raw pies and cookies, all alone. When there are two people, both of them will be involved into food preparation. For example, in the beginning you will be making salads and your buddy can bring a dressing. Later you can learn how to dehydrate crackers and cookies and your buddy will make live pizza or cake. Your buddy-ship will encourage you to learn how to be creative on raw food and will make your life more interesting.

When you don't have a buddy and, say, your friends are gathering for a cooked dinner, you may feel lonely and deprived and tempted. If the same situation is happening but you have a buddy, then a nice lunch or dinner will give you strength. Support helps us to go through the healing crisis without panic. Support helps us to see our own choices and actions in a clearer light. I have seen that people with support were able to stay on raw food for a long time and much easier than people without a support group. Everyone I know who has maintained the raw food lifestyle for several years has had support.

CHAPTER FOURTEEN

Step Seven

I shall find alternative activities or hobbies.

My existence was concentrated around eating. I realized that as soon as I became a raw fooder. When we eat cooked food, we live from meal to meal. We look forward to each snack. We reward ourselves with food. When we want entertainment, we eat. Very often our day is planned like this, breakfast, work, snack, work, lunch, work, snack, work, dinner, TV with a snack, bed. Most people have little or no playing in their life.

When you go on a raw food diet, within a couple of weeks you will notice that your food intake will begin to shrink. In a matter of months your eating could naturally reduce to two meals a day. Then you simply cannot continue to concentrate your life around eating. People who keep concentrating on food begin to feel deprived of joy and fun and eventually get off the raw diet. If you like to eat more than anything else, you better change your hobby.

On raw food your body will require less time for sleep.

Eating less will save you money. You will also have more energy. What are you going to do with all this extra energy, time and money? Please don't say with a smile, "No problem!" Yes, we know how to handle extra money. However, extra energy could make us too nervous. Extra time could lead us into deep depression or into another addiction. Especially when the main pleasure in life, cooked food, is not available. Time and energy are treasures if we use them properly. When you notice that you are eating less, your life cannot concentrate around food any more. You need to find other things and build your life around them.

Think of your life dream that you haven't pursued. In addition to fulfilling your dream, start a couple of hobbies. Pay attention to what other people create out of inspiration. Go to your local YMCA or recreational center for ideas and feel what will attract your heart.

Below are some dreams that people shared at my workshops.

> to do some art work;
> to learn to speak French;
> to write a book;
> to take flute lessons;
> to go on a hike;
> to spend time with children;
> to take yoga classes;
> to play with animals;
> to plant a garden;
> to take Salsa dancing;
> to travel;
> to learn how to sew;
> to scuba-dive.

Every single person has a dream that maybe has been pushed back due to lack of time. Now you can pull out those shining dreams.

I recommend that you also find some form of physical activity for yourself. It will balance the energy of your body and mind. If you had a negative experience with physical exercise in the past, I have good news for you. When you go on raw food, any physical activities are going to be much more pleasant and easy for you to perform. No more stitches or cramps in your side, no more shortage of breath and hardly any injuries. Raw food is still to be discovered by professional athletes.

CHAPTER FIFTEEN

Step Eight

I shall let my higher self lead my life.

We are human beings, spiritual beings. We are not only human bodies. But human bodies are obvious and easy to feel. Our spiritual energy is not as obvious and we begin to ignore it. Our body runs on energy similarly to cellular phones run by electromagnetic waves. We can feel the phone by touch but we cannot feel the electromagnetic waves. If we would ignore these waves, our phones would be useless.

When we are born we are perfectly tuned to our spiritual self. As we grow we learn to behave not as we feel but as we are "supposed" to behave, we attain a second, materialistic personality. This second personality is adjusted to the life in society so well that we use it more and more. Then we begin to identify this second personality with our own self. Finally, we forget who we really are. When we hear someone saying that we are spiritual beings, we feel doubts. Our materialistic self demands proofs. All people are spiritual, nobody is more spiritual than the other. However, most of us forgot about that.

To be driven by a materialistic personality is safer and easier for the career and wealth. There are many other benefits. Only one thing is impossible for the materialistic personality–TO BE HAPPY. Please, don't confuse happiness with pleasure. Pleasure is a short-term emotion. When I buy a new dress or eat a burrito I feel pleasure. Happiness is a spiritual feeling, a permanent state of being.

When we are driven by the materialistic personality we become pleasure-oriented. Pleasures are addictive. That is why in order to quit addictions we need to try our best to tune in to our original spiritual self. How can we do that? There are several ways. None of them guarantees a complete spiritual awakening. But you should be able to feel a connection with your real self.

Spend several days in nature. Your second personality will wither away without worldly support. The energy of nature will interact with your human energy and you will begin to feel happy. Everyone in my family experienced a great happiness, in 1998, when we were hiking the Pacific Crest Trail for six months.

Fast on water for seven days or more. Fasting tremendously increases your energy. You will feel a stronger connection with your spiritual self. Don't fast if you don't know how. Read books on fasting or consult with a specialist before doing so.

Speak sincerely to another human being for two hours or longer. Most people never spoke sincerely in their whole life, so it is not easy. We confuse "sincerely" with "negatively." To speak sincerely doesn't mean to say negative things about yourself, but to share your hidden feelings and passion. Find a good friend who will agree not to judge you for your words and feelings. When you speak sincerely your inner self speaks through your lips. You could be greatly surprised by the power and wisdom in your own words. Also don't confuse sincere talking with friendly chattering.

Communicate with animals. Dogs, horses, cats, goats, dear, etc. don't care how you are dressed, how big your house is and if you are free of debt. But they can feel if you are at peace or angry. They appeal to your human nature and help you to feel connected with your real self.

Play with little children. They are less conditioned and less materialistic. Your second personality can relax around them.

If you meet a person who, you feel, is tuned to his/her spiritual self, being around such a person can awaken your own inner spirit. Similarly, staying around very materialistic people may shut down your spiritual self.

When we are driven by a spiritual personality we feel complete and happy. In this state we simply forget about how we look and what we eat. When we are happy, we concentrate on the most important issues of our life. Food alone is only a small part of our existence. That is why I think to let our higher self lead our life is very essential.

CHAPTER SIXTEEN

Step Nine

I shall make a searching and fearless inventory of the real reasons for seeking comfort and pleasure from cooked foods.

I n this sharing from one of my workshops you can hear the dialogue of other people on the same path. Maybe it will help you to find your own reasons for seeking comfort and pleasure from cooked foods.

Victoria: I would like everyone to share about your real reasons for searching for comfort in food. I want to repeat that when you speak sincerely everybody is interested in listening to you, it triggers in us similarities that we have. We are all different in the ways that we are conditioned, but we are all one in the way we feel. When we are honest, other people, even though they are not ready to express themselves, recognize their feelings in our sharing and they become braver. They might be thinking, "Oh, how dare he? He's saying things that I am afraid to say." After sincere sharing we all feel a relief, we feel happier.

Paul: The food's in my mouth before I even think about it.

Sharon: I want to numb myself out with food. I have eighteen siblings. When I was ten, my mother died from cancer. That's when my desire to numb out started.

Simon: I am addicted to ice cream. It's comforting to reinforce who I think I am, even if I don't really like it. The addiction continues to define me.

Donna: I am working long, hard days. At the end of the day I just want something to give back to me, to fill up the emptiness.

Victoria: Maybe you can try other activities, like growing flowers or horseback riding? You can look forward to them after hard working days, right? Those hard times are still going to be there sometimes. They don't disappear together with cooked food.

Paula: I crave chocolate cake because I am lonely and sometimes I am afraid to stand up for myself and say what I really need.

John: When I need energy I turn to food instead of resting.

Linda: When I was a young child my grandmother nurtured me with food. I realize now that I can nurture myself in a different way.

Mike: I eat from laziness and boredom.

Victoria: Why do you get lazy and bored.

Mike: I live alone.

Victoria: Is living alone enough to be bored? Do you think that relationships will bring health and happiness? If we're lonely alone, we'll be lonely in relationship. Thank you, Mike, for sharing and being open to discussion. So why do we want to eat cooked food?

Simon: Comfort.

Sharon: My growing up years were very structured and I had to eat at certain times. At times I was hungry but I had to wait for dinner. I grew up with fear that there wouldn't be any food when I was hungry. I ate a lot so I wouldn't be hungry.

Julie: I lived in a family that had a lot of control. Food was one way I could have control in my own life. Nobody could take away my food.

Victoria: There is a magic trick in what we are doing now. If you can clearly see the reason why you seek comfort in cooked food and if you can pinpoint what it is, that reason may disappear. Then it would be easier for you to stay on raw food. Please try to see clearly and say why you are looking for comfort in cooked food. Try to be precise and don't be afraid.

John: Whenever I come up against my core emotions or feel vulnerable, I want sugar to numb me out.

Victoria: Do you know how to take care of these feelings without sugar?

John: I want to do it, but I keep postponing until next time.

Victoria: If we don't know how to deal with feeling lonely or sad without cooked food or sugar, we are going to be stuck there. We are trying to figure out for ourselves how we can act as an alternative.

Simon: That is true. Recently I had one "major disappointment" in my life and it caused my returning to cooked food.

Victoria: What are you trying to numb or to comfort? Why do you in particular want something tasty? For comfort? From what? Does everyone understand the question?

We are searching fearlessly and sincerely for the cause of why we search for comfort in food. Like, we don't have enough pleasure from just being alive?

Donna: I'm bored and I want to break out of this routine.

Victoria: Why is your life just routine? Life is beautiful! Turn your life from routine into life. Does what I am saying make sense to you?

Donna: Yes, and sometimes I'm there. I want to find out why I give myself permission to lose it.

Victoria: We are afraid that without food we will feel uncomfortable. Where does this discomfort come from? Fear of what?

Linda: For me, it's fear of emptiness. I do things for others but not for myself, and then I become angry.

Victoria: Thank you for pinpointing it! You are not able to say "no" when you really want to say "no." Then you feel regret, and to comfort that, you eat food. It's important that if you see it now, maybe you won't do it any more. We all resonate with that. Many times when we first hear about raw food we have a deep fear because we think, maybe it won't fulfill us. We are afraid not of the raw food, it doesn't bite. We are afraid of that emptiness.

Mike: Sometimes I use food when I don't want to do something else.

Julie: I agree that I also eat to avoid doing other things I need to do.

Victoria: Interesting that you use the words "things I need to do." Several years ago I decided that I was not going to do anymore of the "need" to do. I decided to only do what I "love" to do. I had to learn to clean my house with love and to have fun while filing some papers. It is something to think about. We can live without the heavy feeling that we must do this and that.

Susan: When I was a young child I had to keep so many secrets. I felt a safety in being mediocre. I don't want to be noticed or to stand out.

Victoria: Can you observe any other ways of dealing with this...feeling safe? Maybe you can speak out all of that to somebody and you will feel safe.

Susan: I have, for ten years in therapy.

Donna: There's so much shame there.

Victoria: Let us look at shame. What is shame? Caring what others think about us. How we feel about ourselves is important. I had so many things I was ashamed of all my life and when I spoke them out, I found out that it was not a big deal. Everybody I talked to said, I feel the same way. There's nothing extraordinary. But I kept secrets for years and my self-esteem was low. I had to pretend I was better because I thought I was bad. Not anymore. Congratulations to you, Susan, on your courage in speaking this in front of thirty people, that's courage.

Sharon: I had a similar experience. That is why I kept weight on for a long time, now I have lost weight since I've been raw. I felt exactly what you are talking about, I was trying to avoid being more attractive, more "out there," it was worth it to go through my fears because I finally can be happy in my body and I can finally get through this stuff instead of running away from it. I have freedom.

Victoria: We have made an inventory and found out that a real reason for seeking comfort from cooked foods is to escape. When we seek pleasure in cooked food or any other addiction, we are seeking escape from loneliness, boredom, low self-esteem, anger, fear and other negative emotions. We escape to something from which we draw pleasure. Clearly seeing the real reasons for searching comfort, we can address our unfulfilled needs directly, instead of numbing them with food.

CHAPTER SEVENTEEN

Step Ten

I shall let my intuition help me.

Why do we need intuition? Aren't we, people, smart without it? Don't we have enough knowledge? Don't we have specialists who can teach us how to stay healthy? Why can't we rely on the information from computers and microscopes? Knowledge can NEVER replace intuition!

Intuition is our natural instinct for survival. Natural instincts of all living things kept our planet in the perfect balance for billions of years. Intuition is a universal law, same as gravity. Paradoxically, we ignore intuition and rely on knowledge. We don't believe in our own intuition. We forgot how to follow it.

A little silly flour worm follows his instinct not to eat rolled oats if they have been steamed. That is the purpose of steaming rolled oats, so that worms would stay away. The flour worm has no knowledge whatsoever, only instinct. He follows his instinct and never eats cooked oats. Flour worms are very healthy. People look at the package of rolled oats to read the nutritional information. Then they eat cooked oats and give it to their children. We wonder why is our health declining? If you really want to become healthy you need to learn how to listen to your intuition. We cannot blindly follow knowledge. When we receive new information we need to test it with our intuition.

Please touch your cheek with your hand. Is it soft? Touch a rug on the floor. Does it feel different? How do you know? You feel that your cheek is soft and the rug is rough. How is your body able to let you know that? Have you ever thought of that? Do you completely trust your hands in dealing with surfaces? Why do you rely on your hands' feelings? Do you just simply trust? What if I bring an expert who wears a $1000 suit and a beautiful tie and speaks very scientifically and prove that the opposite is true. Will you believe him? No? Why? Your body is just a dull matter, as we were told in school.

If we trusted our intuition we would rely on our body. Then we could understand that our body never makes mistakes. Our body is constantly trying to communicate with us by creating certain sensations. When our body lets us know that it is cold we know to put on a sweater. When our body needs rest it creates a sensation of fatigue. When the body needs water it makes us thirsty. If the body is filled with toxins it may reduce our appetite asking for a water fast. Usually we ignore most of our bodily requests. We don't rest when we feel tired, we don't take off high heels when we feel pain in our feet and we don't stop eating when we feel full. That is why we all get sick.

If you would go around asking different people which fruit they would like to eat today, all answers would be different. When you crave a certain fruit or vegetable, that is your body's request for nutrients for today. Tomorrow it might change. Your responsibility is to make sure these orders are satisfied. People who are honoring the body's request are allowed to live longer and healthier lives.

I want to share with you how my family survived in the wilderness thanks to our intuition. When we had just started to hike the Pacific Crest Trail we planned to eat five medjool dates for each of us every day. We were not used to eating only five dates a day. In the first two days we had eaten what we were supposed to eat in ten days and our next package was waiting for us seventy miles ahead at the next post office. We had nothing left to eat except a little bit of oil and a tiny bag of sunflower seeds. So we thought, we will fast. On our fourth day out on the trail we felt very hungry. We observed that the forest is full of animals. There are bears, squirrels, all kind of coyotes, lots of birds, insects and they are all surviving. They're all on a different diet. They're not dying. They have something to eat. All the animals, without coming to my class, know what to eat. If they can survive, we can survive. We began to develop a keen attentiveness to the plants around us. Some of the plants started to look yummy to us. Looking under a rock, something looked thick and juicy, and I tried it ... tasted medicinal ... like perfume. I gave everybody a bag and I said, "When you see something that looks good, just pick it up but don't eat." Soon we each had a big bag of plants. We sat down together and looked at what we had collected. We rubbed the plants with our fingers, smelled the leaves and tasted a little bit on our tongue. We threw away the plants that didn't taste good, were bitter or smelled bad. Now we took the plants that were left and Igor said "I will eat some first and we'll see how I feel and if I don't feel anything bad, then we will all eat it." Igor took a little taste, we waited about thirty minutes and then Igor said, "I'm hungry, let's eat more." So we all ate. The next day as we walked along we filled our bags with whatever edible greens we found. We put our edible greens into a bowl, sprinkled it with sunflower seeds, several drops of oil and tossed it up. It was so delicious. We called our dish the "Hungry Hiker" salad. When we were eating the salad we all agreed that we wanted to continue eating this simply when we got back to town. In the forest we learned to rely on our intuition completely.

We lost our trail many times. After the third month we were not afraid to lose the trail. We were always able to find it. One time we lost the trail and had to travel seven miles to find it. We climbed a 7,000-foot mountain arriving at the snow covered peak. The map showed us that to recover the trail we needed to go straight north from the mountain. However, straight north from the mountain was a deep canyon and it was storming and we all had heavy, wet backpacks. We ignored the map, took the way that felt right, and after six hours we crossed the trail. Our intuition led us through. We met so many different animals along the trail. We were traveling as animals, relying on intuition. We found food when we thought there was none.

On a trail I developed such a keen intuition, I could tell when it was going to rain and when the sun was going to be out. I cannot imagine how I could have lived without this intuition most of my life. I wouldn't trade my intuition for anything in the world.

CHAPTER EIGHTEEN

Step Eleven

Through clarity I will gain happiness.

If you will follow your intuition for a while you might discover that your perception of life is shifting. Many of your favorite beliefs will seem to you as false. Many of your former opinions will seem to lose sense. That won't scare you because in place of your former knowledge the CLARITY will come. Clarity is the biggest gift that we could get.

When we don't have clarity we are trying to accumulate knowledge. Knowledge could never substitute for clarity. I used to believe that "Knowledge is Power." Now I am aware that knowledge is not even information. Knowledge is human's explanation and interpretation of life events. Clarity is a state of mind when we could see life events as they are, without the distortion from knowledge. Very often having knowledge prevents us from gaining a real clarity. Usually we confuse clarity of mind with clear explanation. For example, if I memorized the book *Human Anatomy* and I could explain clearly anything from that book, it doesn't mean at all that I have clarity about how the human body works. We have lots of knowledge and very little clarity. When we don't understand the difference between the two, we prefer to have knowledge rather then clarity. Clarity starts when we begin to follow our intuition. When we follow intuition we are working not against, but with nature. We become co-partners and co-creators with life. That enables us to clearly view the perfect harmony of the universe.

With clarity we can see the spiritual nature of human beings. With clarity we can feel oneness with all living things. With clarity we feel true happiness. When we are truly happy we don't look for pleasures. Only unhappy people are focused on pleasures. Happiness is a part of natural law. To gain clarity practice de-conditioning.

We all have lots of conditioning. To be conditioned means to have firm opinions on everything, to live from the past. To be unconditioned means to live in the present. For example, when we live next to the mountain, at first we admire the beautiful view every minute. After two months we stop noticing that mountain. We become conditioned to know that it's there. Guests notice the mountain because they have a fresh, unconditioned approach to it. We can start noticing the mountain again if we look at it every day with new, fresh eyes. In order to de-condition ourselves we need to be able to see as many conditionings in ourselves as possible. This sharing from my workshop might give you ideas of different conditioning.

Victoria: Please, everybody, share with us an instance where you saw you were conditioned and overcame it. I will start with myself. I used to be conditioned to finish my plate because children in Africa starve.

Linda: I was conditioned that I have to have good grades, otherwise I am a bad person.

Kelly: I used to be conditioned to think that I have to smile to everybody and please them.

Jim: I used to be conditioned to being normal, just fit in.

Laura: I used to be conditioned to being busy all the time.

Mary: I used to be conditioned to pull myself apart from other people, not to share myself with them, not to smile too much, not to get excited.

Sharon: I used to be conditioned to make everything perfect around the house.

Simon: I used to be conditioned to be angry.

Donna: I used to be conditioned to think that men are superior to women.

Val: I used to be conditioned to believe I am fat, ugly and dumb.

Marlene: I used to be conditioned to be poor, to be inexpressive, that I can never have extra money or afford to buy anything rather than necessity.

Shannon: I used to be conditioned to think I am better than others because I am from a wealthy family.

Sam: I used to be conditioned to be a workaholic, I couldn't let myself go on vacation.

Molly: I was conditioned to dress nicely so people would think nicely about me.

Chris: I used to be conditioned to be a pleaser, to think that I am not worth it.

Victoria: Thank you! You see, there are so many conditions that we all have in common. I felt very many of those in me. Conditioning is like chains that don't let us be free. To find those conditionings in us is to our benefit.

CHAPTER NINETEEN

Step Twelve

I shall provide support to other raw fooders.

Please remember the first person in your life who told you about raw food. Who was your first raw food teacher? Think of these people with gratitude. What was special about them? Why did you trust them? Were they patient and empathetic towards you? Did they share a delicious raw meal with you? How would your life be different if you never met them? Now you have finished all 12 steps and became a strong raw fooder yourself. The time has come for you to be patient and empathetic towards other people.

What could be more joyous than to help those looking for better health? Being healthy and being a good example is the best support you can give to other people.

Remember your first raw food potluck. Were you excited by the variety of dishes? Now is your turn to encourage others. Even if you eat simple now, try to bring raw gourmet dishes to potlucks, don't just bring a couple kale leaves or a bowl of fruit. Take your time, spend an extra

$10-$15 and brighten new raw fooder's futures.

I believe that we all are great world teachers. As teachers we have followers. Who do you think would be your students? People who suffer from pain? Your loved ones diagnosed with terminal illnesses? From my experience this is far from the truth. Help those who are directly asking you about your lifestyle. Become their "raw buddy." People who want to know more about a raw food diet don't have anybody else to count on. Spend time with them, talking and listening, preparing meals together, going out to restaurants, and loan them your books. Being a raw buddy is the best support for you too.

How many people do you honestly think you will influence in your life by being a raw fooder? Think of all the people you touch in a day. All your neighbors, relatives, co-workers and people who see you buying and eating healthy food. The cashier at your local store, seeing you buying 50 lb. bags of carrots, asks, "Do you have a horse?" When your children go to school and tell their teacher, "In our family we eat salad every day," don't they influence even the teacher?

What if I had not gone on raw food? What would have happened to all of my students? Many of my former students are now making their living by teaching raw food classes.

You never know when you're going to plant a seed. How many people can you influence in a lifetime? Eventually, I think, the whole planet.

12 STEPS TO RAW FOOD

Step 1 – I admit that I have lost control of my addiction to cooked food and my eating is becoming unmanageable.

Step 2 – I believe that live vegan food is the most natural diet for a human being.

Step 3 – I shall gain necessary skills, learn basic raw recipes and obtain equipment to prepare live food.

Step 4 – I shall live in harmony with people who eat cooked food.

Step 5 – I shall stay away from temptations.

Step 6 – I shall create a support group.

Step 7 – I shall find alternative activities or hobbies.

Step 8 – I shall let my higher self lead my life.

Step 9 – I shall make a searching and fearless inventory of the real reasons of seeking comfort and pleasure from cooked foods.

Step 10 – I shall let my intuition help me.

Step 11 – Through clarity I will gain happiness.

Step 12 – I shall provide support to other raw fooders.

CHAPTER TWENTY

Recipes

Raw Family Green Juice

Blend these ingredients well in a blender:
    1 large bunch kale (chopped)
    2 medium apples (chopped)
    1 lemon with peel (chopped)
    1 cup water

Strain the liquid through a nut milk bag or sprouting bag.
Serves: 3-4 people.

Borscht

Blend these ingredients well in a blender or Vita-Mix:

  2 cups water
  3 beets
  1 small root ginger (slice it first)
  3-4 large cloves garlic
  6-7 bay leaves

Pour the mixture into a big bowl.

Blend the following ingredients for a short time (about 30 seconds):

  2 cups water
  2 carrots
  2 stalks celery
  2 tablespoons apple cider vinegar
  3-4 oranges, peeled with the seeds out
    (seeds will make very bitter taste)
  1 tablespoon honey
  1 cup olive oil
  sea salt to taste

Add $^1/_2$ cup walnuts and blend on low speed very quickly, so they break in small pieces but not blended. Pour in the same bowl and stir.

Dice or grate:

  $^1/_4$ head cabbage
  1-2 carrots
  1 bunch parsley

Add grated ingredients to the blended mixture. Stir and serve. *Serves 7-10.*

Un - Chicken Noodle Soup

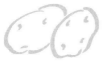

Blend together **very** well for 1-2 minutes:
>   2 cups water
>   1/2 cup coconut (shredded, unsulphered)

Add the following and blend for about 1 minute:
>   2 cups celery (chopped)
>   2 tablespoons Bragg's Liquid Aminos
>   1 clove garlic
>   pepper to taste, if desired

Pour into a large bowl and add:
>   1 medium carrot (grated)
> $^1/_4$ of a bunch parsley (chopped)
>   2 medium raw potatoes, grated or
>   processed with Saladacco
>   sliced mushrooms (optional)

Serves 7.

Generic Recipe for Chowder

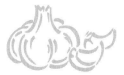

Blend 1 cup coconut with 1 cup of water for 1 minute in Vita-Mix or 2 minutes in regular blender.

Add 1 cup cashews and blend for another 1/2 minute.

Add the rest of the following and blend well:

> 1 cup water
> ¹/₂ cup extra virgin olive oil
> 1 teaspoon honey
> 1 cup chopped celery
> hot peppers to taste
> 2-5 cloves garlic

Now you have plain chowder. *Pick the flavor:*
For clam-chowder taste add: dulce flakes
For broccoli: chopped broccoli
For mushroom: your favorite mushrooms, dry or fresh
For tomato: chopped tomato
For carrots: grated carrots
For corn: cut corn off the cob or use frozen corn
For pea: fresh or frozen peas
Your own creation . . .
Sprinkle with dry parsley flakes before serving.

Note: this soup will become warm because of much blending. It's still raw. (Just don't let it become hot!) Warm soups are comforting in the cold winter time. Serves 5.

Chili

Blend the following ingredients in a blender:

    1 cup water
    2 cups fresh tomatoes (chopped)
    $^1/_2$ cup dates or raisins
    $^1/_2$ cup extra virgin olive oil
    1 cup sun-dried tomatoes
    1 cup dehydrated mushrooms
    1 cup chopped celery
    salt or Bragg's Liquid Aminos to taste
    1-2 tablespoons spaghetti seasoning
    1-2 tablespoons juice of lime or lemon
    hot peppers to taste
    2-5 cloves garlic
    1 bunch basil

Add $^1/_2$ lb. of bean, pea, or lentil sprouts. Don't blend! Sprinkle with dry parsley flakes before serving.

Note: chili will become warm because of much blending. It's still raw. (Just don't let it become hot!) Warm dishes are comforting in the cold wintertime. Serves 5-7.

Gazpacho

Blend the following ingredients in a blender until smooth:
> $^1/_2$ cup water
> $^1/_4$ cup extra virgin olive oil
> 5 large ripe tomatoes
> 2 cloves garlic or spicy pepper to taste

1 tablespoon raw honey (dates or raisins work just as good)
> $^1/_4$ cup lemon juice
> $^1/_2$ teaspoon of sea salt
> 1 bunch fresh basil

Now you have the gazpacho liquid.
Cut the following vegetables into $^1/_4$ inch cubes:
> 1 large avocado
> 1 medium bell pepper
> 5 sticks celery
> 1 small onion

Mix all ingredients in bowl and sprinkle with chopped parsley. *Serves: 4-5*

Generic Recipe for Dressing

Blend the following until smooth in a blender:

    Oil (any good oil, such as sesame,
        olive, safflower). Use enough
        to cover the blades of a blender.

  1 teaspoon honey (or any other
      natural sweetener, like raisins, banana,

  2 tablespoons fresh lemon juice (or lime
      juice or apple cider vinegar)

$^{1}/_{3}$ cup water

1 cup chopped or 1 bunch herbs - preferably
    fresh! (one or more of: celery, parsley,
    cilantro, basil or any other)

spice to taste (garlic, mustard, ginger,
    jalapeno, etc.)

$^{1}/_{3}$ cup seeds or nuts (the most common are
sunflower seeds and tahini; also: walnuts,
pumpkin seeds, almonds, etc.)

$^{1}/_{2}$ teaspoon, salt (sea salt, kelp, dulce, Bragg's
Liquid Aminos) or to taste or no salt at all

Don't be afraid to improvise. You may sometime add more
liquid, or skip one ingredient completely. If it tastes good,
put it in. Good luck! *Serves 7-10.*

Igor's Crackers

Grind 2 cups of flaxseed in a dry Vita-mix container.
Blend together:

> 1 cup water
> 1 large onion (chopped)
> 3 stalks of celery (chopped)
> 4 cloves of garlic (medium)
> 2 tomatoes (optional)
> 1 teaspoon caraway seed
> 1 teaspoon coriander seed
> 1 teaspoon Celtic salt

Mix ground flaxseed in blended mix by hand.

Cover the dough with a cheesecloth or a towel and let sit in a
bowl at a warm room temperature overnight to ferment
slightly.

Using a spatula, spread on teflex dehydrating sheets. Divide
into squares of desired size. Dehydrate only until dry, but not
crispy if you want it to taste like bread. Or dry it well for
crispy crackers to keep them for a couple of months. *Makes
25-32 crackers.*

Valya's Raw Bread

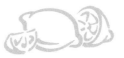

1 cup ground flaxseeds
1 cup kamut sprouted for 1 day
1 cup walnuts soaked overnight
1 cup chopped celery
2 teaspoons caraway seeds soaked overnight
2 tablespoons coriander
1 big onion
$^1/_2$ cup water
$^1/_2$ cup olive oil
$^1/_2$ cup raisins
Juice of half a lemon
1 teaspoon salt

Blend soaked walnuts, kamut and onion in the food processor until finely chopped, transfer to a bowl and mix with the ground flaxseeds. Next blend celery, olive oil, raisins, and water in a blender. Combine both mixtures. Add the salt, coriander, lemon juice, and caraway and mix thoroughly. Shape the mixture into small loaves and place on a teflex dehydrator tray, make sure to decorate your loaves with crushed nuts or poppy seed. Place in the dehydrator at 100 degrees, for about 24-36 hours. You may need to flip the bread after approximately 12-15 hours so that both sides dry evenly. *Makes 5-7 loafs.*

Live Gardenburgers

Grind 1 lb. of your favorite nuts in a food processor. Combine the following ingredients and put through a Champion Juicer with the blank plate in or grind in a food processor:

> 1 lb. carrots
>
> 1 medium onion
>
> 1 tablespoon sweetener (honey, very ripe banana, raisins)
>
> 1 tablespoon oil
>
> 1-2 tablespoons poultry seasoning (or other seasoning)
>
> sea salt to taste
>
> 2-3 tablespoons nutritional yeast (optional)

If the mixture is not firm enough, add one or two of the following thickeners: dill weed, dried garlic, dried onion, dried parsley flakes, nutritional yeast, psyllium husk powder, ground flaxseeds.

Form into balls, cutlets, or fillets and sprinkle with paprika a little before serving.

Note: If you want "fishburger" add seaweed (dulse, kelp, nori) to the mixture. *Serves 10.*

Portabella Mushroom Burger

Grind 1 lb. of your favorite nuts in a food processor. Combine the following ingredients and put through a Champion Juicer with the blank plate in or grind in a food processor:

>1 lb. carrots
>1 medium onion
>1 tablespoon sweetener (honey, very ripe banana, raisins)
>1 tablespoon oil
>1-2 tablespoons poultry seasoning (or other seasoning)
>sea salt to taste
>2-3 tablespoons nutritional yeast (optional)

If the mixture is not firm enough, add one or two of the following thickeners: dill weed, dried garlic, dried onion, dried parsley flakes, nutritional yeast, psyllium husk powder, ground flaxseeds.

Form into 10 burgers. Slice 2 large, ripe tomatoes and 1 large red onion. Have the following ready:

>10 small (or 5 large) portabella mushroom caps
>10 leaves fresh spinach

Assemble mushroom burgers as follows: put mushroom cap upside down on a plate, put spinach leaf on it, put burger on spinach, put slice of tomato on burger, put slice of onion on tomato. You may secure your "sandwich" with toothpicks. *Serves 10.*

Live Fries

Slice 1 lb. jicama so it looks like French fries.

Combine in a bowl with:
> 1 tablespoon onion powder
> 2 tablespoons extra virgin olive oil
> sea salt to taste
> 1 tablespoon paprika

Serves 5.

Live Pizza

Crust:

Grind 2 cups of flaxseed in a dry Vita-mix container.
Blend together:
> 1 cup water
> 1 large onion (chopped)
> 3 stalks celery (chopped)
> 2 tomatoes (medium)
> 4 cloves garlic (medium)
> 1 teaspoon Celtic salt

Mix ground flaxseed into blended mix by hand. Spread on dehydrating sheets with a spatula. Divide into squares of desired size. Dehydrate only until dry, but not crispy.

Topping:

Blend the following ingredients with as little water as possible:

1 lb. of any nuts
$^{1}/_{2}$ cup sun-dried tomatoes
$^{1}/_{2}$ cup raisins
juice of 1 medium lemon
2 tablespoons olive oil
1 tablespoon dry basil

Pour in a bowl. Add:

1 tablespoon dry onion
1 tablespoon dry garlic
2-3 tablespoons nutritional yeast
1 tablespoon miso

Mix well.

Making pizza:

Spread topping on squares of crust.
Decorate with grated yams, sliced cherry tomatoes, sliced mushrooms, sliced olives and chopped parsley. *Makes nine "slices" of pizza.*

Nori Rolls

Paté mixture:

$^1/_2$ cup walnuts

2 cups sunflower seeds soaked overnight

3 cloves garlic

1 cup chopped celery

1 $^1/_2$ teaspoons salt

$^1/_3$ cup olive oil

$^1/_2$ cup lemon juice

1 teaspoon curry powder (or your favorite seasoning)

Additional ingredients:

Slice the following into thin, long strips:

Half an avocado

Half a large bell pepper

2 green onions

5 raw nori sheets

Blend all the paté ingredients in a food processor until creamy.

Spread the pate onto a sheet of nori and add the thinly sliced vegetables. Roll up tight in nori sheet. Note: to make the nori sheets stick better you can moisten them a little with water, lemon, tomato or orange juice. Let the nori rolls sit for 10 minutes and then begin slicing them into 2 inch slices. *Makes 10-15 nori rolls.*

Un–Spaghetti

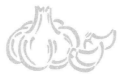

Shred or use Saladacco to create thin noodle-like-strands of butternut squash. Sprinkle with paprika and oil before serving. Decorate with fresh parsley.

Tomato Basil Sauce:

Blend 2 cups fresh chopped tomatoes.
Add the following ingredients and blend:

        2-4 cloves garlic
        $^3/_4$ cup chopped fresh basil
        juice of 1 medium lemon
        2 tablespoons olive oil
        4 dates (or some raisins)
        1 cup sun-dried tomatoes

Serves 7.

Nut or Seed Cheese

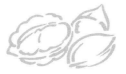

2 cups any nuts or seeds soaked overnight
1 ¹/₂ cup pure water

Soak the nuts and seeds in pure water overnight. Drain and
rinse the nuts and seeds. Put into blender with one cup of
pure water and blend well to break the nuts down into a fine
cream. Pour into sprout bag. Hang the sprout bag over a sink
or bowl (to pour off the whey) and let ferment at room temperature for approximately 8-12 hours.

Transfer cheese to a bowl, mix with your favorite seasonings
and stir well.

Yield 1 pint. Keeps for at least 7 days in a covered container
in the refrigerator.

To flavor seed cheese you may use any combination of the
following: garlic, lemon juice, chopped fresh cilantro, Bragg's
Liquid Aminos or Nama Shoy, curry powder, chopped or dry
parsley, chopped or dry dill, sun-dried tomatoes, chopped
scallions, basil, olive oil, sea-salt.

Valya's Spicy Almond Cheese

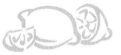

Mix the following ingredients in a bowl:

> 2 cups of pulp from almond milk (pulp should not be sweet)
> $^1/_4$ cup olive oil
> $^1/_2$ cup lemon juice
> $^1/_2$ teaspoon of salt
> $^1/_4$ cup fresh or dried dill weed
> $^1/_2$ cup diced onions
> $^1/_2$ cup diced red bell pepper

Decorate with cherry tomatoes. *Serves 4.*

Pecan Paté

Mix the following ingredients in food processor until finely
chopped:

> 3 cups raw pecans soaked over night
> $^1/_2$ cup of dates
> 3 cloves garlic (spicy pepper works great)
> $^1/_4$ cup lemon juice
> $^1/_4$ cup olive oil
> $^1/_4$ cup fresh cilantro
> $^1/_2$ teaspoon sea salt

Use paté to stuff bell peppers, cabbage leaves, nori rolls, etc.
Serves: 5-6 people

Sunny Spread

> $^1/_2$ cup walnuts
> 2 cups sunflower seeds soaked overnight
> 3 cloves garlic
> 1 cup chopped celery
> 1 $^1/_2$ teaspoons salt
> $^1/_3$ cup olive oil
> $^1/_2$ cup lemon juice
> 1 tablespoon dry basil

Blend ingredients in food processor until smooth. Be creative
and serve on cracker, rolled up in a cabbage leaf or stuff a
bell pepper. *Serves 12.*

Sergei's Hummus

Blend the following ingredients in a food processor:

2 cups garbanzo beans sprouted for 1 day

¹/₂ cup extra virgin olive oil

1 cup tomatoes (chopped)

1 cup celery (chopped)

salt or Bragg's Liquid Aminos to taste

1-2 tablespoons (dry) or 1 cup (fresh)
dill or basil

1-2 tablespoons lime or lemon juice

hot peppers to taste

2-5 cloves garlic

Sprinkle with dry parsley flakes before serving.
Serves 5-7.

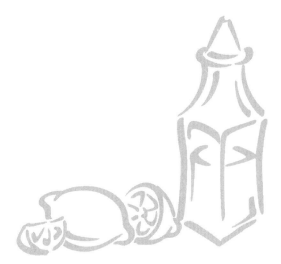

Generic Cake Recipe

Crust:
Combine the following ingredients, mixing well:

        1 cup ground nuts, seeds or grains
        1 tablespoon oil
        1 tablespoon honey

Optional:

        $^1/_2$ cup chopped or crushed fresh fruits or berries or $^1/_2$ cup dry fruits, soaked for 1-2 hours, then ground
        1 teaspoon vanilla
        $^1/_2$ teaspoon nutmeg
        $^1/_2$ cup raw carob powder
        peel from 4 tangerines, well ground

If mixture is not firm enough, add psyllium husk or shredded coconut. Form into crust on a flat plate.

Topping:
Blend the following ingredients well; add water with a teaspoon if needed:

        $^1/_2$ cup fresh or frozen fruit
        $^1/_2$ cup nuts (white nuts look pretty)
        $^1/_2$ cup olive oil
        2-3 tablespoons honey
        juice of 1 medium lemon
        1 teaspoon vanilla

Spread evenly over the crust. Decorate with fruits, berries and nuts. Give your cake a name. Chill.

Nuts, seeds and grains: almonds, walnuts, filberts, cashews, pine nuts, pecans, sunflower seeds, flaxseed, sesame or tahini, oat flour or rolled oats, buckwheat, kamut or barley.

Dried fruits: pitted prunes, raisins, apricots, dates, figs or currants.

Fresh fruits and berries: strawberries, apples, bananas, blueberries, pineapple, mangoes, apricots, raspberries or cranberries.

Serves 12.

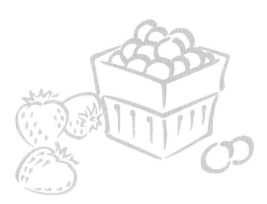

Sergei's Young Coconut Dream Cake

This cake won a contest at the Portland Raw Food Festival.

Crust:

> 1 cup raw unsoaked walnuts
> $^1/_2$ cup of your favorite pitted dates
> $^1/_2$ cup young coconut water
> 4 tablespoons raw carob
> 1 small papaya

Blend the walnuts and dates in a food processor until the mixture is smooth. Mix in the carob and the coconut water. Spread one layer of crust out on a plate. Place sliced papaya on top of first layer. Place second layer on top.

Icing:

> 1 cup young coconut meat
> Water, enough to blend into thick topping
> 1 tablespoon honey

Blend all the ingredients in a vita-mixer. Spread icing on cake. Decorate with fruit slices and nuts.

Un-Chocolate Cake

Crust:
Combine the following ingredients, mixing well:
> 1 cup ground nuts
> 1 tablespoon oil
> 1 cup raisins
> 1 cup raw carob powder
> 1 teaspoon Frontier's butterscotch flavor
> 1 teaspoon vanilla
> $^1/_2$ teaspoon nutmeg, Nama Shoyu or Bragg's
>   Liquid Aminos
> peel from 4 tangerines, well ground
> 1 cup prunes soaked for 1-2 hours ground

Form into one-inch layer on a flat plate. Spread ground prunes between layers (form as many layers as you want).

Topping:
Blend the following ingredients well; add water with a teaspoon if needed:
> 1 cup ripe avocado meat
> 1 teaspoon olive oil
> 3 tablespoons honey
> juice of 1 medium lemon
> 1 teaspoon vanilla
> 4-5 tablespoons carob powder

Spread evenly over the crust, or squeeze using decorating bag. Decorate with fruits, berries and nuts. Chill. *Serves 12.*

Macadamia Date Pie

Crust:

> 4 cups macadamia nuts
> 2 cups dates
> juice of one orange
> 1 teaspoon salt
> $^1/_4$ teaspoon of butterscotch or vanilla extract

Blend macadamia nuts in food processor until they are finely chopped and transfer to a bowl. Next blend the dates and orange juice in a food processor and add to the macadamia mix. Mix thoroughly together with salt and butterscotch extract.

Spread the crust out thinly on a normal size plate. Finely slice bananas or your favorite fruit and spread on top of the macadamia date crust. Next cover the fruit with another layer of the macadamia date mixture.

Decorate the pie with thinly sliced oranges and nuts or your favorite fruits. *Serves 8-12 people.*

Sergei's Amazing Truffles

1 cup raw unsoaked walnuts
$^1/_2$ cup of your favorite pitted dates
$^1/_4$ cup young coconut water
4 tablespoons of raw carob

Blend the walnuts and dates in a food processor until the mixture is smooth.

Mix the carob and coconut water. Shape the mixture into small balls and roll the balls in carob, decorate with your favorite fruit. *Makes 8-12 truffles.*

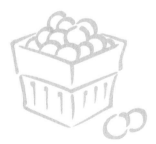

Alla's Cranberry Scones

2 cups grated apples
2 cups carrot pulp after you make carrot juice
2 cups raisins or chopped dates
1 cup cranberries (fresh or dry)
2 tablespoons honey
2 cups almonds ground
1 cup flaxseed blended with 1 cup water
$1/2$ cup olive oil

Mix with hands. You have to experiment to get the consistency desired. Drop by spoonfuls onto teflex sheets.

Dehydrate at 105-115 degrees for several hours. Approximately 4 hours on one side, flip for 3 hours on opposite side.

Makes 24 scones.

Sergei's Butternut Squash Cookies

4 cups peeled butternut squash chopped into
medium sized chunks
1 cup raisins
juice of one orange
$^1/_2$ teaspoon nutmeg
1 teaspoon cinnamon
3 tablespoons raw honey

Blend the chopped squash in a food processor and transfer
into a bowl. Next blend the raisins and the orange juice in a
food processor and add to the squash mixture. Add the rest
of the ingredients into the bowl and mix thoroughly.

Use an ice cream scoop and scoop the mixture onto a dehydrator tray, flatten each cookie untill they are one inch thick.
Set the dehydrator for 100 degrees and leave in for 12–15
hours.

Makes 7-11 cookies.

Valya's Almond Orange Cookies

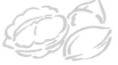

Blend the following ingredients in a food processor until they are finely chopped:

> 4 cups raw almonds soaked overnight
> 2 cups raisins
> $^1/_2$ cup orange peel
> 2 medium oranges whole
> $^1/_2$ teaspoon salt
> 2 apples

When all the ingredients are finely processed, use a spatula to spread cookie mixture onto a dehydrator tray at 115 degrees for 20 hours or until dry. Decorate each cookie with sliced nuts or raisins.

Yields 10-12 cookies.

Macadamia Date Cookies

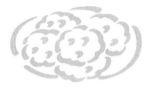

4 cups macadamia nuts
2 cups dates
juice of one orange
1 teaspoon salt
$^1/_4$ teaspoon of butterscotch or vanilla extract

Blend macadamia nuts in food processor until fine and transfer to a bowl. Next blend the dates and orange juice in a food processor and add to the macadamia mix. Mix thoroughly together with salt and butterscotch extract.

Scoop the mixture onto teflex dehydrator trays and decorate with pine nuts. Set at 100 degrees and dehydrate for 12-15 hours. Serve warm.

Makes 7-12 cookies.

Sesame Cookies

A fabulous way to use all leftover sesame pulp after making sesame milk.

> 5 cups sesame seed pulp
> 2 cups raisins
> 3 tablespoons raw honey
> juice of one orange

Blend raisins and orange juice in food processor until mixture is finely pureed. Add to a bowl with the sesame seed pulp. Add honey and mix thoroughly. Spread the mixture onto teflex dehydrator sheets and using a spatula cut into squares. Sprinkle with poppy seeds and set in the dehydrator at 100 degrees. Dehydrate for 12-15 hours or until dry. *Makes 15-20 cookies.*

Morning Cereal

> Soak 1 cup of oat groats overnight
> Blend with $^3/_4$ cup water
> Add $^1/_4$ cup of dates without pits or raisins and blend
> Add 1 tablespoon of your favorite oil (optional)
> Add salt to taste (optional)

Garnish with fresh fruits and berries before serving. *Serves 3-4.*

Buckwheat Millet
Morning Cereal

Soak the following overnight:
>   1 $1/2$ cups millet
>   2 cups buckwheat
>   1 cup coarsely chopped hazelnuts

Additional ingredients:
>   1 cup raisins
>   3 tablespoons honey
>   1 teaspoon cinnamon

Using a rolling pin, flatten the millet and the buckwheat. Transfer the grains into a bowl and add the crushed hazelnuts. Add the rest of the ingredients and mix thoroughly.

Spread the mixture evenly onto a dehydrator sheet. It is important to avoid spreading the mixture too thin or too thick. Set the dehydrator for 100 degrees and dehydrate until the cereal is completely dry, which will take between 10–12 hours. Serve with nut milk.

Makes 3-6 servings.

Sergei's Favorite Smoothie

Blend all ingredients in a blender until smooth:
>   2 oranges (peeled)
>   2 frozen bananas (other frozen fruit is
>   optional)

Place the oranges towards the bottom of blender to make enough liquid to blend the frozen bananas.
Decorate with fresh strawberries!
Serves 2-3 (until you get addicted, then it only serves 1).

Nut or Seed Milk

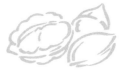

>   1 cup any nuts or seeds soaked overnight
>   2 cups pure water
>   1 tablespoon honey or 2-3 dates
> $1/4$ teaspoon Celtic salt (optional)

Blend all ingredients in a blender thoroughly until smooth.
Strain mixture through a sprout bag. Pour into a jar. *Serves 4.*

Un-Chocolate Almond Milk

1 quart almond milk
$^1/_2$ cup dates
1 young coconut (meat and water)
2 tablespoons raw carob powder
1 raw vanilla bean

Blend well in a blender. Serve chilled. *Serves 5-7.*

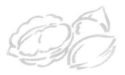

Nut Milk Shake

Blend the following ingredients in a blender until smooth:
3 cups almond milk
$^1/_2$ cup fresh or frozen strawberries
1 medium orange (peeled)
1 fresh or frozen banana
2 tablespoons honey or $^1/_4$ cup of pitted dates
$^1/_4$ teaspoon sea salt
1 vanilla bean
$^1/_2$ cup of ice (ice is not necessary if you use
frozen fruit)
Serves 4-5.

Nut or Seed Yogurt

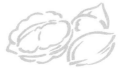

1 cup any nuts or seeds soaked overnight
1 1/2 cup pure water

Blend nuts with water in a blender thoroughly until smooth.
Keep adding water, until you have the consistency of heavy
cream. Strain mixture through a sprout bag. Pour into a jar
and cover with a cheesecloth for the transfer of air and gases.
Set your jar in a warm place where the yogurt temperature
can heat up to 90-100 degrees. It will be ready in approximately 6 to 12 hours or when it tastes tart and sour.

Nut and seed yogurts can be made from sesame seeds,
almonds, pecans, hazelnuts, cashews, sunflower seeds and any
other nuts, seeds or their combinations. You may play with
taste by adding honey, lemon juice, sea salt, vanilla, or other
flavors. The longer your yogurt will stay in a warm place the
stronger and more sour it will become.

Suggested combinations for making delicious yogurt:

Cashew	Sesame and almond
Cashew and sesame	Sunflower and almond
Cashew, almonds	Pecans and almonds
and sesame	Walnuts and pine nuts
Cashew and sunflower	Sesame and hazelnuts

Creative Health Institute

'The Wheatgrass Place'
Creative Health Institute teaches the
Dr. Ann Wigmore program of Living Foods.

Creative Health Institute celebrated its 25th Anniversary in October 2001. Founded by Donald O. Haughey, the facility was inaugurated by Dr. Ann Wigmore, who often taught here during her life. Our programs are designed to follow her teachings as best we can, as articulated in her books *Why Suffer?* and *Be Your Own Doctor.*

Our learn-by-doing program includes the use of wheatgrass to detoxify and facilitate rejuvenation, indoor/organic gardening, body-hygiene, enzyme nutrition, composting, sprouting, meal preparation, energy soup, and gentle exercise focused on stretching and breathing.

This program is conducted as a detoxification and rebuilding system of nutrition, which participants take home and incorporate with their lifestyle. This experience is foundational to establishing a living-foods wellness way of life.

Thousands from around the world have traveled to Creative Health Institute, to learn prevention of illness and reversal of disease with the Living Foods Lifestyle. Come, join us in a great journey into healthful living during a time it is so needed on our beautiful planet.

 Creative Health Institute
www.creativeinstitute.us

Phone: (517) 278-6260 • e-mail: info@creativeinstitute.us
112 W. Union City Rd., Union City, Michigan 49094

THE VALUE OF SUPPORT

by Raw Seattle Support Groups
www.rawseattle.org

Using the 12 Steps to Raw Food that have been developed by Victoria Boutenko, Raw Seattle has formed two weekly support groups. Much of the Raw Seattle community began living the raw food lifestyle as a result of her influence, and many of the members of our support groups began participating as soon as they finished Victoria's class. The support groups have matured into a mini-community of adventurous, caring and enthusiastic humans exploring the boundaries of their known world and creating entirely new ways of living life. In several other communities of the Northwest where Victoria has taught, students have also formed support groups that meet on a regular basis.

The transition from the cooked food world to the raw food lifestyle has been very challenging for many of our members. Those who rely on will power alone to leave the addictions of the cooked food way of life often cannot make a permanent change. The support group has provided a natural framework of assistance in achieving a 100% raw food lifestyle. This facilitated environment of structure and confidentiality allows group members to share from the heart with sincerity what is true for them according to their direct, personal experience.

We, in Seattle, are eager to share our story in order to inspire other communities to form their own support groups. If we can be of assistance, please contact www.rawseattle.org. The calendar will list the most appropriate contact person for the support group at that time.

AUTHOR BIO

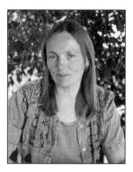

Victoria Boutenko teaches classes on Raw Food at Southern Oregon University. Her classes are highly in demand. As a result of her teachings, many raw food communities, have been formed through the world.

When Victoria is not teaching or writing she enjoys hiking, swimming and biking with her raw family in Ashland Oregon.

The transformation of Victoria's family to raw food is described in their book "Raw Family."

Order Form

for books by

Raw Family Publishing

Online orders: www.RawFamily.com

E-mail: Victoria@rawfamily.com

Postal orders:

Raw Family Publishing

P.O. Box 172

Ashland, OR 97520

Please send (   ) copies of *12 Steps to Raw Food* @ $11.95

Please send (   ) copies of *Raw Family* @ $11.95

Please send (   ) copies of *Eating Without Heating* @ $11.95

Please send (   ) copies of videotape "Raw Gourmet Dishes Simplified"

(Victoria teaches how to prepare 14 basic raw dishes) 2003 @ $19.95

Shipping and handling: $3.50 for the first book or tape and $1.00 for each additional

Payment: Check or money order

Total $_____

Name:_____

Address:_____

City:_____State:_____Zip:_____

Telephone:_____

E-mail address:_____

Wholesale discounts available on large quantities.

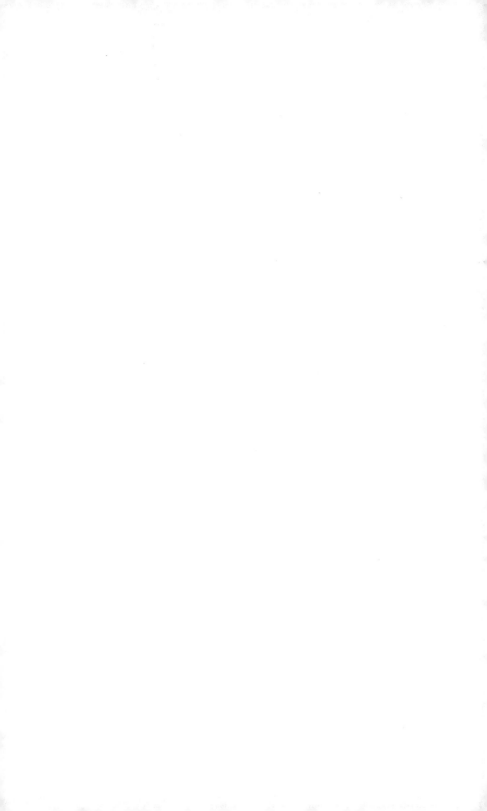